Molecular Docking and Molecular Dynamics

Edited by Amalia Stefaniu

Published in London, United Kingdom

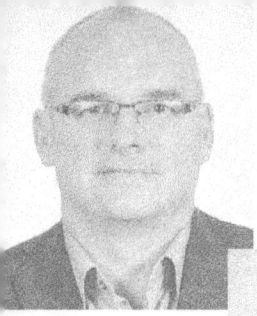
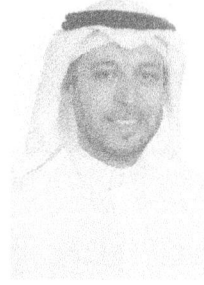
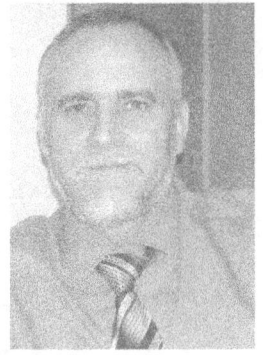
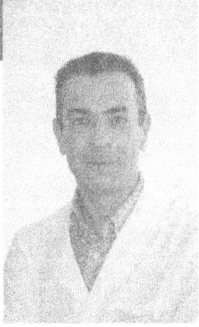
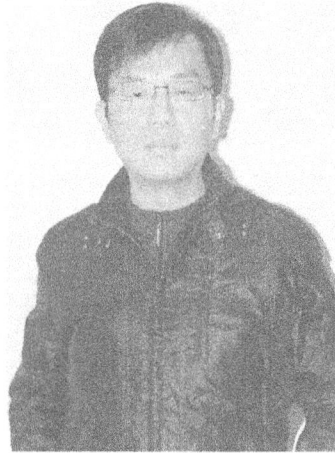
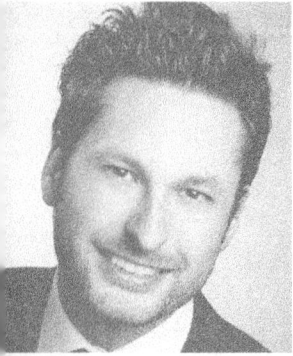
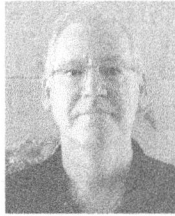

IntechOpen

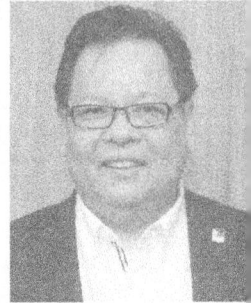
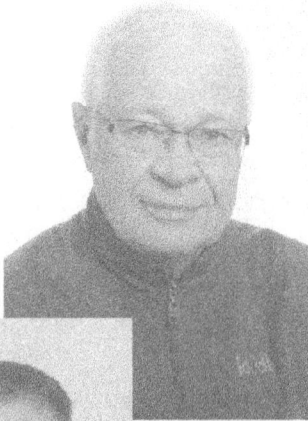
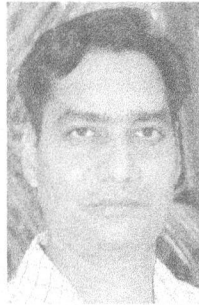
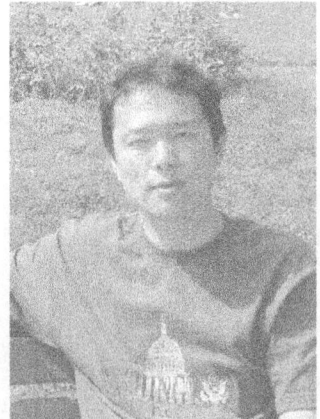
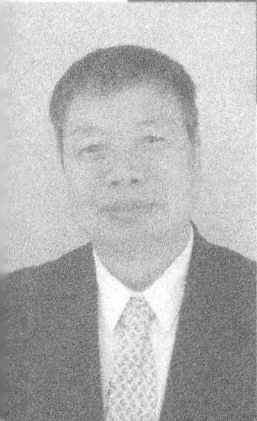
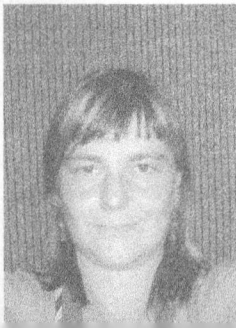

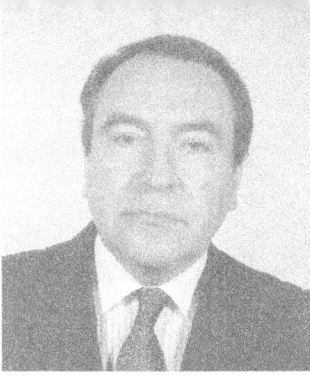

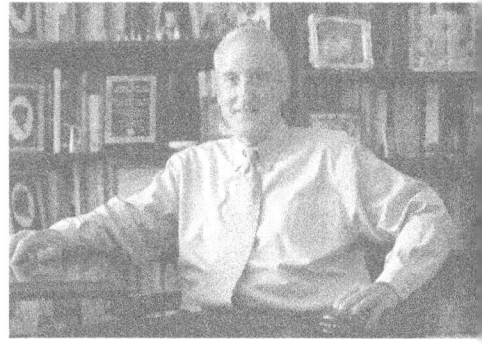

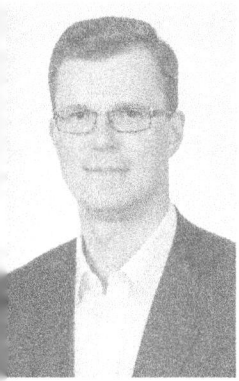

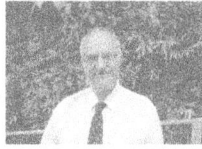

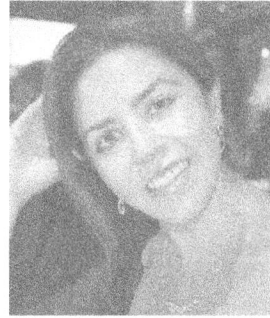

Supporting open minds since 2005

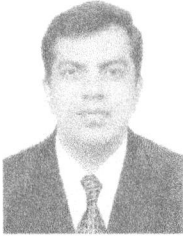

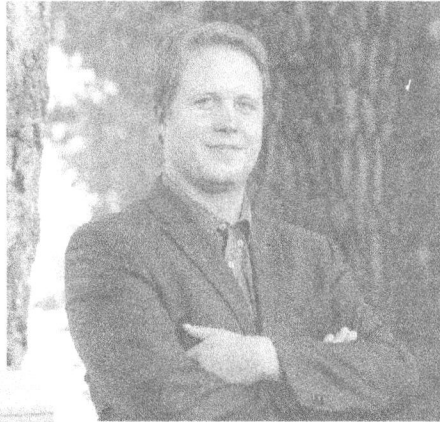

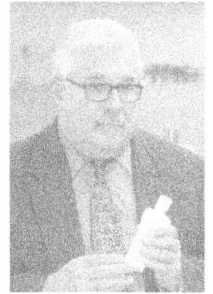

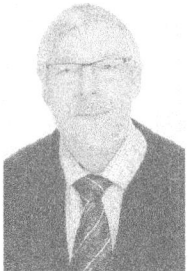

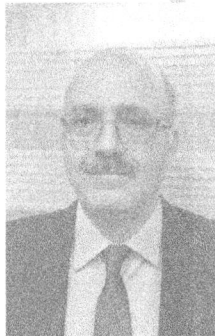

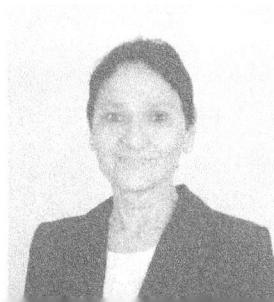

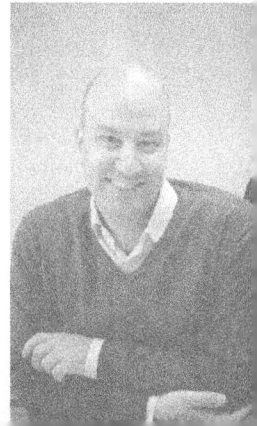

Molecular Docking and Molecular Dynamics
http://dx.doi.org/10.5772/intechopen.77898
Edited by Amalia Stefaniu

Contributors
Evren Gundogdu, Emre Ozgenc, Emine Selin Demir, Meliha Ekinci, Makbule Asikoglu, Derya Ozdemir, Lucia Pintilie, Amalia Stefaniu, Xiongwu Wu, Bernard Brooks, Sentot Joko Raharjo, Stefan Paula, Adam McCluskey, Jennifer R Baker, Xiao Zhu

Notice
Statements and opinions expressed in the chapters are these of the individual contributors and not necessarily those of the editors or publisher. No responsibility is accepted for the accuracy of information contained in the published chapters. The publisher assumes no responsibility for any damage or injury to persons or property arising out of the use of any materials, instructions, methods or ideas contained in the book.

First published in London, United Kingdom, 2019 by IntechOpen
IntechOpen is the global imprint of INTECHOPEN LIMITED, registered in England and Wales, registration number: 11086078, 7th floor, 10 Lower Thames Street, London, EC3R 6AF, United Kingdom
Printed in Croatia

British Library Cataloguing-in-Publication Data
A catalogue record for this book is available from the British Library

Additional hard and PDF copies can be obtained from orders@intechopen.com

Molecular Docking and Molecular Dynamics
Edited by Amalia Stefaniu
p. cm.
Print ISBN 978-1-78984-091-9
Online ISBN 978-1-78984-092-6
eBook (PDF) ISBN 978-1-78985-262-2

We are IntechOpen,
the world's leading publisher of
Open Access books
Built by scientists, for scientists

4,500+
Open access books available

118,000+
International authors and editors

130M+
Downloads

Our authors are among the

151
Countries delivered to

Top 1%
most cited scientists

12.2%
Contributors from top 500 universities

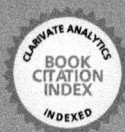

CLARIVATE ANALYTICS
BOOK
CITATION
INDEX
INDEXED

WEB OF SCIENCE™

Selection of our books indexed in the Book Citation Index
in Web of Science™ Core Collection (BKCI)

Interested in publishing with us?
Contact book.department@intechopen.com

Numbers displayed above are based on latest data collected.
For more information visit www.intechopen.com

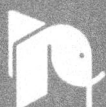

Meet the editor

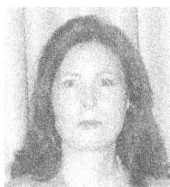

Amalia Stefaniu has a background in chemical engineering, acquiring her bachelor's degree at Politehnica University of Bucharest, Faculty of Engineering, in Foreign Languages. She followed up her postgraduate academic studies in Drugs and Cosmetics with a master's degree in Biotechnologies and Food Safety. She completed her PHD in Exact Sciences, Chemistry Domain, in 2011 at University Politehnica of Bucharest, Faculty of Applied Chemistry and Materials Science, Department of Inorganic Chemistry, Physical Chemistry and Electrochemistry. She joined the National Institute for Chemical Pharmaceutical Research and Development, Bucharest, in 2001, where she worked as Chemical Research Engineer in Pharmaceutical Biotechnologies. Her current position is senior research scientist. Her researche focuses on properties prediction, mathematical modeling, molecular docking, and therapeutic compounds design.

Contents

Preface

The rise of chemical information and development of structure databases, as well as the need for new therapeutic agents or improved specific materials with controlled properties, has led to the development of chemoinformatic tools. These tools can be used to design new molecules and to model their chemical and/or biochemical environment and interactions. Molecular docking and dynamic simulations are such approaches whose methodologies have evolved in terms of accuracy. Thus, today researchers benefit from important *in silico* studies and new opportunities to identify and propose new hit molecules further to chemical synthesis or isolation from vegetal materials, as first step in the introduction in therapeutic practice of new agents.

This book clearly explains the principles of molecular docking and molecular dynamics. It includes examples of algorithms and procedures proposed by different software programs for visualizing and identifying potential interactions in complexes of biochemical interest.

The book is organized into six chapters, each one discussing different molecular simulation methodologies and providing concrete examples of complex interactions. In each chapter, the authors provide an overview of the treated subject, a description of the methodologies used, and a discussion of the results.

Chapter 1 is an introductory chapter, familiarizing the reader with basic principles and terminology of docking and dynamic simulations.

Chapter 2 addresses one of the most common cancer diagnoses in women, breast cancer. The authors use homology modeling, ligand docking, and molecular dynamic simulations to explore aryl hydrocarbon receptor (AhR) structure and to identify its suitable binding site for some aromatic acrylonitrile ligands, potential drug candidates in therapeutics of breast malignancies. The work highlights the usefulness of homology modeling in cases when the protein domain of interest is not yet described and characterized by X-ray crystallography. The employed methodologies could serve to assess other compounds' potency as anticancer agents, in virtual screening, before chemical synthesis, evaluation, and pre-clinical trials.

In Chapter 3, the authors report results of docking simulations using quinolone derivatives to evaluate their potential antitumoral and antimycobacterial activity, compared to the standard therapeutic compounds of topotecan and levofloxacin.

Chapter 4 gives a detailed overview of molecular recognition occurring in protein-ligand complexes, based on various type of interactions and other factors (surrounding solvent, ionization effects, conformational changes, entropy, desolvation, etc.) important for the understanding of biological functions and therapeutic action. The authors underline the importance of proper selection of modeling protocols to obtain desired accuracy. A virtual screening of sesquiterpenoid alcohols against cyclooxygenase isoenzymes is realized in an attempt to design and develop new nonsteroidal anti-inflammatory drugs.

In Chapter 5, the authors describe a new implemented methodology to perform protein-protein docking by introducing map objects. This approach should solve the problem of molecular description of very large biomolecular assemblies. Authors use as an example a T-cell receptor variable domain to illustrate the modeling process with map objects and acetylcholine binding protein (ACHBP) to construct its pentamer using protein-protein docking methodology. Their molecular modeling results can be further extended to large biomolecular assemblies.

Chapter 6 refers to theoretical aspects of computational methodologies regarding the design and development of radiopharmaceuticals and their specific applications, especially in assessment of their structure details and parameters. The authors highlight the possible advantages of the use of such methods to increase the personalization of dosimetry in nuclear medicine administration.

These structure-based design approaches offer students and researchers a general idea of the current state-of-the-art docking and dynamic simulations tools and their capability to predict ligand binding modes in various complexes and assemblies. I hope readers will find these studies instructive and inspirational for further research ideas, contributing to the inter-disciplinary efforts in bio- and chemoinformatics, pharmacology, and medicine.

Amalia Stefaniu
National Institute for Chemical - Pharmaceutical
Research and Development – ICCF Bucharest,
Department of Pharmaceutical Biotechnologies,
Laboratory of Molecular Design and Molecular Docking,
Bucharest, Romania

Introductory Chapter: Molecular Docking and Molecular Dynamics Techniques to Achieve Rational Drug Design

Amalia Stefaniu

Molecular docking and molecular mechanics simulations are important approaches to achieve a rational drug design or a chemical process modeling. It goes to deep molecular insights as structures and mechanisms helping researchers to characterize various conformations and molecular interactions in terms of energy and binding affinities, giving the possibility to search among dozens, hundreds of real or imaginary compounds, the most suitable for a precise, well-defined purpose. The biochemical purpose derives from the chosen macromolecular target, protein, or enzyme. Starting from a known substance with a known mechanism of action and biological activity, we can imagine other related compounds as drug candidates with better efficacy and fewer side effects. These in silico methods help us to identify and select among large compound libraries the most suitable therapeutic agent before even starting its chemical synthesis. That can be called virtual chemistry before reaction tube. It is very convenient, reducing the consumption of chemical reagents, preclinical, clinical trials, and time.

The purpose of this book project is to clearly explain the principles of molecular docking and molecular dynamics, with examples of algorithms and procedures proposed by different software programs for small molecule-protein or protein-protein complexes of medical or materials sciences interest.

Molecular docking studies provide us an overview of type of interactions occurring in ligand (small molecule)-protein or protein-protein complexes and rank the candidate poses by their affinity scoring function.

The concept of molecular recognition of ligand at the protein/enzyme active site, classically named "lock and key," has been extended at "hand and glove," considering the protein flexibility and reciprocal adaptability between the receptor and ligand [1].

Molecular dynamics simulations explore extrinsic surface and bulk properties of various forms of pharmaceutically active molecules to aid the selection of a successful candidate. It involves accurate evaluation of binding pathways, kinetics, and thermodynamics of ligands in different solvents.

Both these computer-aided drug design (CADD) methods lead to ligand identification and optimization, favoring rapid development of pharmaceutical compounds.

1. Molecular docking approaches and challenges

Different software algorithms use various approaches such as rigid protein or flexible protein, rigid receptor, soft receptor, flexible side chains, induced fit, or multiple structure algorithms [2].

The steps for conducting molecular docking studies are:

- Ligand preparation consists in generation, optimization, and analysis of its 3D structure. Among multiple conformers, the most stable, as lowest energy, can be used for docking simulations. An aspect to be considered is the fact that in physiological media, the ligand appears ionized. The effect of solvation due to the surrounded water molecules must be solved. The presence of active site water molecules influences the docking pose of the ligand and makes questionable the accuracy of the method [2]. Three-dimensional structures of small ligand molecules are available in virtual databases such as Cambridge Structural Database (CSD), Available Chemical Directory (ACD), MDL Drug Data Report (MDDR), or National Cancer Institute Database (NCI).

- Receptor preparation. The use of a rigid target protein will conduct a single conformation of the receptor. Flexible protein involves different conformations to bind the ligand. Often the site water molecules are removed before performing a docking simulation.

Protein Data Bank (https://www.rcsb.org/) provides various solved 3D structures of protein, protein fragments, nucleic acids, and protein-ligand complexes. The assemblies are characterized by X-ray crystallography, nuclear magnetic resonance (NMR), infrared spectroscopy, and or/electron density and are available as PDB files format. This online tool allows us to explore and analyze the structures or to compare any protein in the PDB archive, including support for rigid-body and flexible alignments.

Also, for simulation the optimized ligand structure must be imported and used in the docking software as *.pdb or compatible file.

- Identify the binding site: This step plays a key role in structure-based drug design. It can be determined experimentally or computationally. Some software are created to identifying and analyzing binding sites and predicting receptor druggability [3].

- Dock ligands: Different algorithms are used, fragment-based algorithms, genetic algorithm, Monte Carlo algorithms, and molecular dynamics protocols.

- Docking validation and results analysis: For validation, the software must reproduce the real binding site that was founded and characterized by X-ray crystallography or NMR techniques. To dock ligand similar derivative structures, the same binding site is used, and different conformation dues to rotations around flexible bond are performed for each new structure. The results conduct to predicting preferential binding orientation and the strength of binding affinity, interactions (type, strength, bond length); the conformations are ranked by mean of scoring functions [or root-mean-score deviation (RMSD)]. Furthermore, the stability of receptor-ligand complexes is assessed, and ligand/pharmaceutical small compound druggability is evaluated.

Pharmaceutical applications

- Exploring DNA binding properties of some malignant tumor chemotherapeutic agents [4–7] (to identify the DNA binding site, to predict interactions between potential therapeutic compound and DNA, to assess the stability of DNA-complexes, and to establish correlations between structure and cytotoxicity).

- In silico modeling as attempts to find new efficient therapeutic compounds against pathogens, causative agents of infectious disorders, antitubercular drugs [8–11], antibiotics agents against Escherichia coli [12–14], Pseudomonas aeruginosa [14–16], Staphylococcus aureus [13, 14, 16–19], Bacillus cereus [13, 16], Klebsiella pneumoniae [13], or others.

The computational findings must be completed and confirmed by biological assays to determine in vitro activity, by measuring minimum inhibitory concentration against tested microorganisms.

Molecular dynamics (MD) simulations are useful approaches when analysis of thermodynamic and kinetic properties of ligand-binding events is required to consider. Besides, MD has become effective tools used to modeling chemical processes and to evaluating different parameters of materials in different media (water or gas): velocity direction of removal of material electrical discharge machining (EDM) [20], indentation [21], wear and friction [22], nano-cutting [23], and laser machining [24].

Author details

Amalia Stefaniu
National Institute for Chemical, Pharmaceutical Research and Development, Romania

*Address all correspondence to: astefaniu@gmail.com

IntechOpen

References

[1] Sledz P, Caflisch A. Protein structure-based drug design: From docking to molecular dyamics. Current Opinion in Structural Biology. 2018;**48**:93-102

[2] Elokely KM, Doerksen RJ. Docking challenge: Protein sampling and molecular docking performance. Journal of Chemical Information and Modeling. 2013;**53**(8):1934-1945J. DOI: 10.1021/ci400040d

[3] Halgren TA. Identifying and characterizing binding sites and assessing druggability. Journal of Chemical Information and Modeling. 2009;**49**(2):377-389. DOI: 10.1021/ci800324m

[4] Agarwal S, Chadha D, Mehrotra R. Molecular modeling and spectroscopic studies of semustine binding with DNA and its comparison with lomustine–DNA adduct formation. Journal of Biomolecular Structure & Dynamics. 2015;**33**(8):1653-1668

[5] Subhani S, Jamil K. Molecular docking of chemotherapeutic agents to CYP3A4 in non-small cell lung cancer. Biomedicine & Pharmacotherapy. 2015;**73**:65-74. DOI: 10.1016/j.biopha.2015.05.018

[6] Cathcart J, Pulkoski-Grossa A, Cao J. Targeting matrix metalloproteinases in cancer: Bringing new life to old ideas. Genes and Diseases. 2015;**2**(1):26-34

[7] Pirvu L, Stefaniu A, Neagu G, Albu B, Pintilie L. In vitro cytotoxic and antiproliferative activity of Cydonia oblonga flower petals, leaf and fruit pellet ethanolic extracts. Docking simulation of the active flavonoids on anti-apoptotic protein Bcl-2. Open Chemistry. 2018;**16**(1):591-604

[8] Nunn CM, Djordjevic S, Hillas PJ, Nishida C, Ortiz de Montellano PR. The crystal structure of Mycobacterium tuberculosis alkylhydroperoxidase Ahpd, a potential target for antitubercular drug design. The Journal of Biological Chemistry. 2002;**277**:20033-20040. DOI: 10.1074/jbc.M200864200

[9] Salunke SB, Azad AK, Kapuriya NP, Balada-Llasat JM, Pancholi P, Schlesinger LS, et al. Design and synthesis of novel anti-tuberculosis agents from the celecoxib pharmacophore. Bioorganic & Medicinal Chemistry. 2015;**23**(9):1935-1943. DOI: 10.1016/j.bmc.2015.03.041

[10] Tiwari R, Möllmann U, Cho S, Franzblau SG, Miller PA, Miller MJ. Design and syntheses of anti-tuberculosis agents inspired by BTZ043 using a scaffold simplification strategy. ACS Medicinal Chemistry Letters. 2014;**5**(5):587-591. DOI: 10.1021/ml500039g

[11] Umesiri FE, Lick A, Fricke C, Nathaniel TI. Boronic-aurone derivatives as anti-tubercular agents: Design, synthesis and biological evaluation. Medicinal Chemistry. 2015;**5**:437-441. DOI: 10.4172/2161-0444.1000297

[12] Cheng K, Zheng Q-Z, Qian Y, Shi L, Zhao J, Zhu H-L. Synthesis, antibacterial activities and molecular docking studies of peptide and Schiff bases as targeted antibiotics. Bioorganic & Medicinal Chemistry. 2009;**17**(23):7861-7871

[13] Gullapelli K, Brahmeshwari G, Ravichander M, Kusuma U. Synthesis, antibacterial and molecular docking studies of new benzimidazole derivative. EJBAS. 2017;**4**(4):303-309

[14] Pintilie L, Stefaniu A, Nicu AI, Maganu M, Caproiu MT. Design, synthesis and docking studies of some novel fluoroquinolone compounds with antibacterial activity. Revista de Chimie. 2018;**69**(4):815-822

[15] El-Attar MAZ, Elbayaa RY, Shaaban OG, Habib NS, Wahab AEA, Abdelwahab IA, et al. Design, synthesis, antibacterial evaluation and molecular docking studies of some new quinoxaline derivatives targeting dihyropteroate synthase enzyme. Bioorganic Chemistry. 2018;**76**:437-448

[16] Srivastava R, Gupta SK, Naaz F, Singh A, Singh VK, Verma R, et al. Synthesis, antibacterial activity, synergistic effect, cytotoxicity, docking and molecular dynamics of benzimidazole analogues. Computational Biology and Chemistry. 2018;**76**:1-16. DOI: 10.1016/j.compbiolchem.2018.05.021

[17] Barakat A, Al-Majid AM, Al-Qahtany BM, Ali M, Teleb M, Al-Agamy MH, et al. Synthesis, antimicrobial activity, pharmacophore modeling and molecular docking studies of new pyrazole-dimedone hybrid architectures. Chemistry Central Journal. 2018;**12**(1):29-42. DOI: 10.1186/s13065-018-0399-0

[18] Pintilie L, Stefaniu A, Nicu AI, Caproiu MT, Maganu M. Synthesis, antimicrobial activity and docking studies of novel 8-chloro-quinolones. Revista de Chimie. 2016;**67**(3):438-445

[19] Pintilie L, Stefaniu A, Nicu AI, Negut C, Tanase C, Caproiu MT. Design, synthesis and molecular docking of some oxazolidinone compounds. Revista de Chimie. 2018;**69**(11):2981-2986

[20] Yue X, Yang X. Study on the distribution of removal material of EDM in deionized water and gas with molecular dynamics simulation. 18th CIRP Conference on Electro Physical and Chemical Machining (ISEM XVIII) Procedia CIRP 42. 2016. 691-696

[21] Cheong WCD, Zhang LC. Molecular dynamics simulation of phase transformations in silicon monocrystals due to nano-indentation. Nanotechnology. 2000;**11**:173-180

[22] Maekawa K, Itoh A. Friction and tool wear in nano-scale machining-a molecular dynamics approach. Wear. 1995;**188**(1-2):115-122

[23] Zhang L, Zhao HW, Dai YYH, Du XC, Tang PY, et al. Molecular dynamics simulation of deformation accumulation in repeated nanometric cutting on single-crystal copper. RSC Advances. 2015;**5**:12678-12685

[24] Shih C-Y, Shugaev MV, Wu C, Zhigilei LV. Generation of subsurface voids, incubation effect, and formation of nanoparticles in short pulse laser interactions with bulk metal targets in liquid: Molecular dynamics study. Journal of Physical Chemistry C. 2017;**121**(30):16549-16567. DOI: 10.1021/acs.jpcc.7b02301

Binding of Chlorinated Phenylacrylonitriles to the Aryl Hydrocarbon Receptor: Computational Docking and Molecular Dynamics Simulations

Stefan Paula, Jennifer R. Baker, Xiao Zhu
and Adam McCluskey

Abstract

The development of ligands capable of binding to the aryl hydrocarbon receptor (AhR) and hijacking its signaling pathway is of potential use for the design of novel agents against breast cancer. To guide the synthesis of new compounds and characterize their binding to the AhR, we employed homology modeling, ligand docking, and molecular dynamics simulations. As there is currently no crystallographic information available for the structure of the AhR's ligand-binding PAS-B domain, a homology model was developed. The location of the binding site was identified by scanning the model for concave areas and comparing them to known ligand-binding sites in proteins related to the AhR, such as the CLOCK:BMAL1 transcriptional activator complex and the hypoxia-inducible factor-2α (HIF-2α). Docking of several chlorinated phenylacrylonitriles was performed with the modeling suite MOE, identifying π-π stacking, hydrophobic, and van der Waals interactions as the driving forces for binding, an observation consistent with the hydrophobic nature of the site. Molecular dynamics simulations with one of the compounds for 100 ns verified the overall stability of a docking-predicted pose and revealed the presence of interacting water molecules in the vicinity of the ligand. Given the buried location of the ligand in the core of the receptor, this observation was somewhat unexpected, but it explained a slight shift of the ligand pose seen during the simulation.

Keywords: homology model, molecular dynamics, MOE, ligand-binding interactions, docking, breast cancer, aryl hydrocarbon receptor

1. Introduction

The aryl hydrocarbon receptor (AhR) is a member of the basic helix-loop-helix/Per-ARNT-SIM (bHLH/PAS) transcription factor family [1–4]. In its inactive state, the AhR resides in the cytosol of the cell as a complex with a number of other proteins. This complex ensures the stability of the AhR in a high-affinity ligand-binding form and prevents the premature translocation of the receptor. Upon binding of a ligand, it dissociates from these proteins and travels to the cell nucleus, where it binds to DNA xenobiotic response elements (XREs). This in turn induces the expression of several cytochrome P450 enzymes and a sulfotransferase (typically SULT1A1) that contain XREs in their promotor sequence. These enzymes then initiate the oxidative breakdown of the offending compound.

The AhR pathway has a number of roles, including as a modulator of viral immunity and the correct functioning of the female reproductive system. Its most well-known role is a mechanism by which cells defend themselves against the toxic effects of polycyclic and polyhalogenated aromatic hydrocarbons, such as the Seveso toxin dioxin (**1**) (**Figure 1**) [5, 6].

Hijacking of the pathway is based on the use of compounds capable of activating the pathway and then converting into highly reactive species such as nitrenes once being targeted by the metabolic enzymes. This process ultimately leads to DNA damage and the death of the affected cell (**Figure 2**) [7].

It has been noted that the AhR detoxification process involves the active transport of a ligand, e.g., **1–4**, but not the inhibition of the AhR, which would result in a buildup of toxic materials within the cell. This hijacking of the AhR signaling pathway has been proposed as a novel strategy for designing a new class of drugs against breast cancer [1, 8]. Several compound classes, such as the aromatic acrylonitriles, have shown promise in cell-based assays, displaying remarkable potency and selectivity for breast cancer cells [9, 10]. Two reported AhR ligands, Aminoflavone (**2**) and Phortress (**3**) (**Figure 3**), have progressed to clinical trials, demonstrating the clinical applicability of this approach [11, 12]. Based on this, we have postulated that the AhR is a promising target in the development of breast cancer-specific drugs. In particular, our early studies have demonstrated activity against triple negative breast cancer cell lines [9, 10, 13]. This makes AhR ligands, including the aromatic acrylonitriles, promising candidates for further development into novel agents against breast cancer, that act by a hitherto unexploited mechanism of action.

Here, we demonstrate the use of computational tools for the elucidation of the interactions between the AhR and a targeted selection of chlorinated phenylacrylonitriles. The methods employed include homology modeling, molecular docking, and molecular dynamics (MD) simulations to model the structure of the ligand-binding domain of the AhR, identify its ligand-binding site, characterize critical ligand/

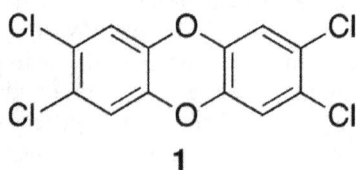

1

Figure 1.
The aryl hydrocarbon receptor ligand 2,2,6,6-tetrachlorodioxin (1).

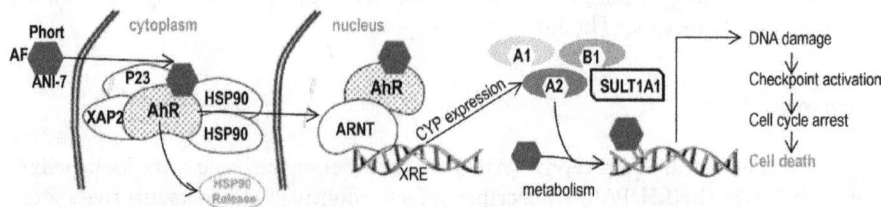

Figure 2.
The AhR pathway showing ligand binding, nuclear translocation, CYP1 activation, metabolism, and cell death. AF = Aminoflavone (2), Phort = Phortress (3), and ANI-7 = (Z)-2-(3,4-dichlorophenyl)-3-(1H-pyrrol-2-yl) acrylonitrile (4) (see Figure 3 for details).

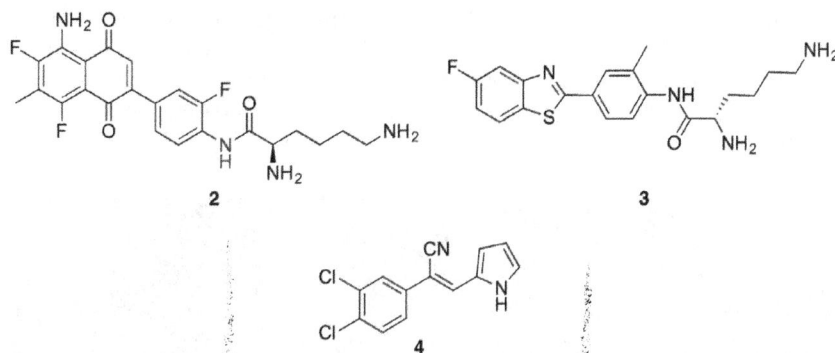

Figure 3.
The known AhR ligands, Aminoflavone (2) and Phortress (3), that have proceeded to clinical trials for the treatment of cancer and our recently reported lead AhR ligand, ANI-7 (4) [13].

receptor interactions, and study the time-dependent behavior of a ligand bound to the AhR. The results illustrate the value of computational tools for revealing the potential binding mechanism of these compounds to their target and for guiding the synthesis of novel compounds with improved properties.

2. Homology model

The sequence of the human form of the AhR was downloaded from the NCBI website (access code: NP_001612.1). Since only the ligand-binding PAS-B domain was of interest to our study, the sequence was appropriately truncated before Pro275 and after Lys397. A search in the modeling suite MOE's structural database for suitable templates returned the structures of 4F3L [14], 3RTY [15], and 2KDK [16] as the best matches. Of these, only 4F3L, a murine transcriptional activator complex, provided complete coverage of the PAS-B domain with a sequence identity of 24.4% and a sequence similarity of 48.0% (**Figure 4**). Only three indels were noted in the

```
NP_00161  ..............................................................
4F3L.A    GAVEEDDKDKAKRVSRNKSEKKRRDQFNVLIKELGSMLPGNARKMDKSTVLQKSIDFLRK

NP_00161  ..............................................................
4F3L.A    HKETTAQSDASEIRQDWKPTFLSNEEFTQLMLEALDGFFLAIMTDGSIIYVSESVTSLLE

NP_00161  ..............................................................
4F3L.A    HLPSDLVDQSIFNFIPEGEHSEVYKILSTHLLESDSLTPEYLKSKNQLEFCCHMLRGTID

NP_00161  ..............................................................
4F3L.A    PKEPSTYEYVRFIGNFKSLTSVSTSTHNGFEGTIQRTHRPSYEDRVCFVATVRLATPQFI

NP_00161  PSILEIRTKNFIFRTKHKLDFTPIGCDAKGRIVLGYTEAELCTRGSGYQFIHAADMLYCA
4F3L.A    KEMCTVEEPNEEFTSRHSLEWKFLFLDHRAPPIIGYLPFEVLGT.SGYDYYHVDDLENLA

NP_00161  ESHIRMIKTGESGMIVFRLLTKNNRWTWVQSNARLLYK..NGRPDYIIVTQRPLTDEEGT
4F3L.A    KCHEHLMQYGKGKSCYYRFLTKGQQWIWLQTHYYITYHQWNSRPEFIVCTHTVVSYAEVR

NP_00161  EHLRK
4F3L.A    AE...
```

Figure 4.
Alignment of the target sequence of the human form of the AhR (NP_00161) with the sequence of a murine transcriptional activator complex, 4F3L.

alignment—deletions of positions 361 and 362 in the target sequence and an insertion in position 308. The absence of major gaps in the alignment is favorable for the development of homology models as it reduces the need for loop modeling and grafting, which can be challenging [17]. Model development based on the alignment in **Figure 4** was performed using MOE's default settings.

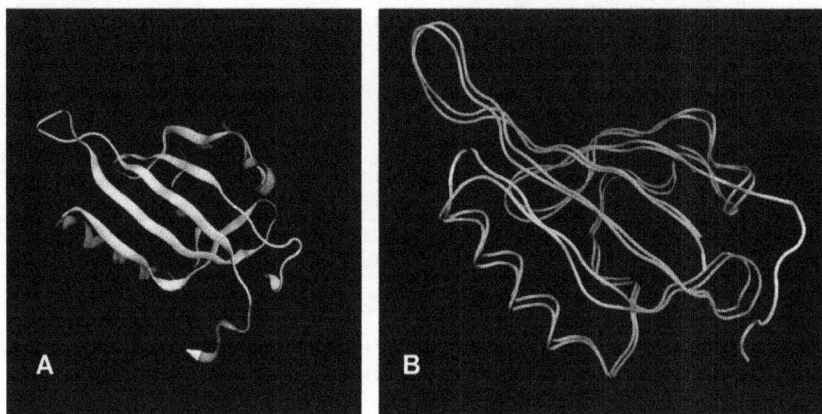

Figure 5.
(A) Homology model for the AhR colored by secondary structure. (B) Comparison of backbone traces of homology models obtained by using the MOE modeling suite (template 4F3L) and the automated SWISS-MODEL server (template 5SY7). Coloring is according to RMSD between the two structures (green—yellow—red, in order of increasing deviation), showing very good agreement between the two models. The model obtained from the SWISS-MODEL server had a somewhat longer sequence, resulting in the gray loops at the termini that have no counterpart in the MOE model.

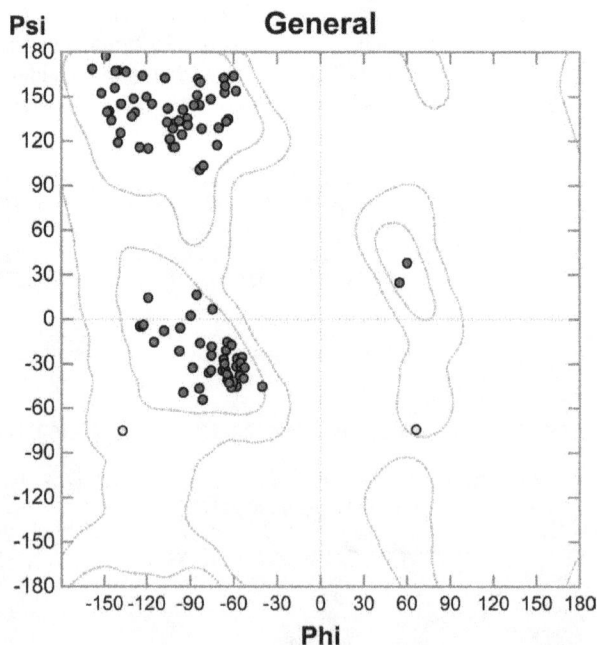

Figure 6.
Ramachandran diagram for the homology model for the AhR. Green (•) symbols represent torsion angles in favored regions, whereas yellow (○) symbols represent angles in allowed regions. No entries are present in the "forbidden" areas.

The resulting homology model of the AhR (**Figure 5A**) was subjected to a number of quality tests, such as an analysis of the Ramachandran diagram (**Figure 6**) and an inspection of observed bond lengths, bond energies, and torsion angles. No abnormalities that would have questioned the quality of the model were detected.

An additional check of the model's reliability was carried out by submitting the PAS-B sequence to the automated server SWISS-MODEL [18]. The returned homology model was superimposed to the model obtained from MOE. Even though the new model was derived using a different template (5SY7, an NPAS3-ARNT complex) [19], a very good agreement between the backbones of the two structures was observed (**Figure 5B**), which further instilled confidence in the accuracy of the model.

3. Computational ligand docking

Before ligands could be docked into the homology model of the AhR, the exact location of the binding site had to be identified. We subjected the homology model to a binding site search, a feature implemented in MOE that screens the surface of a protein for concave areas capable of binding small molecules. Two areas large enough to accommodate a typical AhR ligand were detected: one on the surface and another one in the core of the receptor. To decide which of these two sites was more realistic, the crystal structures of the ligand/receptor complexes 3F1O [20], 3H7W [21], and 3H82 [21], all of which are proteins related to the AhR, were superimposed onto the homology model. As shown in **Figure 7**, all three ligands were found in an area equivalent to the binding site located at the center of the protein (**Figure 5**). To facilitate a convenient designation of the binding site for the subsequent docking runs, the ligand of 3F1O—N-[2-nitro-4-(trifluoromethyl)phenyl]morpholin-4-amine (5)—was copied into the file of the homology model as a point of reference.

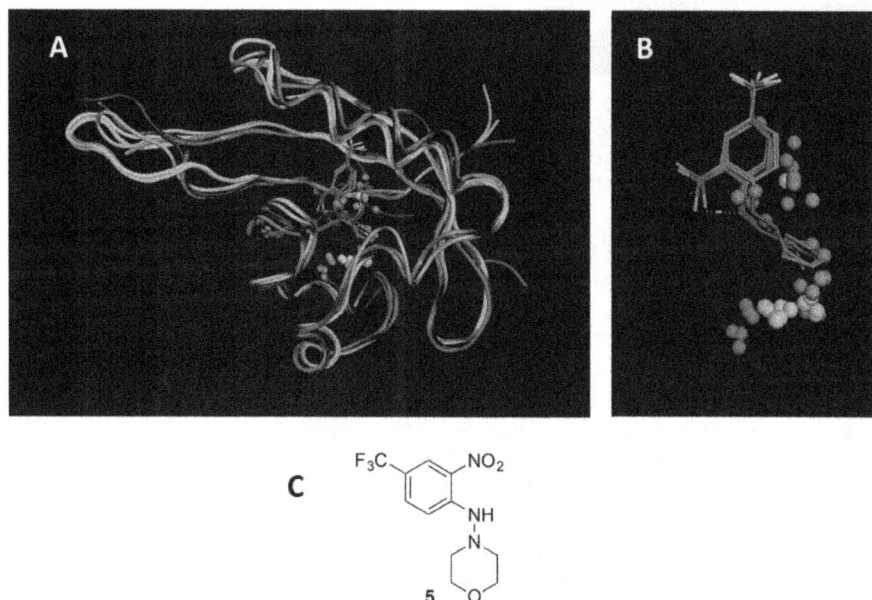

Figure 7.
(A) Superposition of protein/ligand complexes related to the AhR onto the homology model of the AhR. Spheres delineate the putative binding site predicted by MOE that coincides with the position of the ligands seen in the crystal structures. (B) A closeup view of the ligand 5, overlaid with the spheres depicting the binding site predicted by MOE. (C) The chemical structure of the ligand of 3F1O—N-[2-nitro-4-(trifluoromethyl)phenyl]morpholin-4-amine (5).

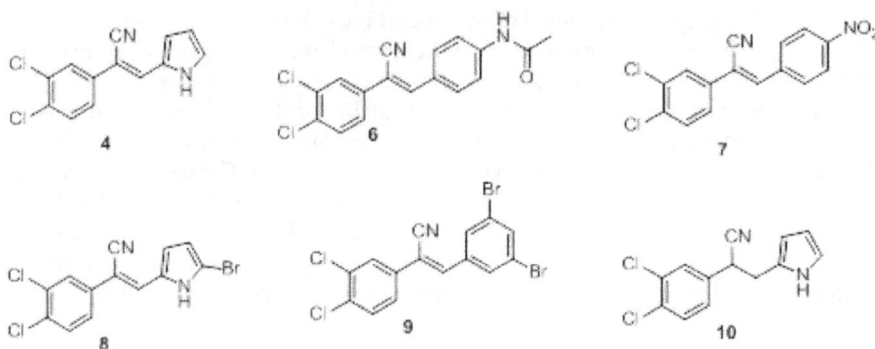

Figure 8.
Structures of six dichlorophenylacrylonitriles (4, 6–10) used for docking.

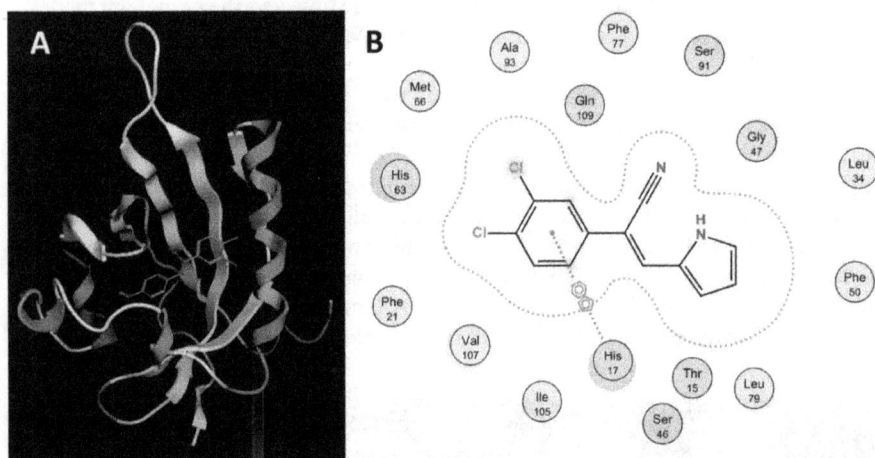

Figure 9.
(A) 3D representation of dichlorophenylacrylonitrile 7 docked into the binding site of the AhR, illustrating the central nature of the site. (B) Interaction diagram of the pyrrole ligand ANI-7 (4), showing π-π-interactions, hydrophobic contacts, and shape complementarity as the driving forces for ligand binding.

To analyze the utility of this model for further drug development, the structures of a representative ensemble of six dichlorophenylacrylonitriles with known bioactivities (**Figure 8**) were modeled in MOE. Their conformational energies were minimized by molecular mechanics in conjunction with the MMFF94x force field. Docking was performed with the default settings of MOE, utilizing a flexible ligand and a mostly static receptor structure and defining the binding site by a position equivalent to that of the ligand present in 3F1O. The top-scoring pose for each ligand was considered for further analysis.

As shown in **Figure 9**, the docked compounds occupied a narrow and mostly hydrophobic site in the core of the AhR. Almost all ligands in the pool engaged with the AhR in a similar fashion, binding in comparable binding poses and exhibiting similar ligand/receptor interactions. Key hydrophobic contacts were observed between nonpolar regions of the ligands and the side chains (Phe21, Leu34, Phe50, Met66, Leu79, Ala93, Ile105, and Val107). Moreover, the ligand phenyl ring engaged in π-π stacking interactions with the ring of His 17. In addition, the tight fit between the ligands and the site suggested the presence of extensive favorable van der Waals interactions.

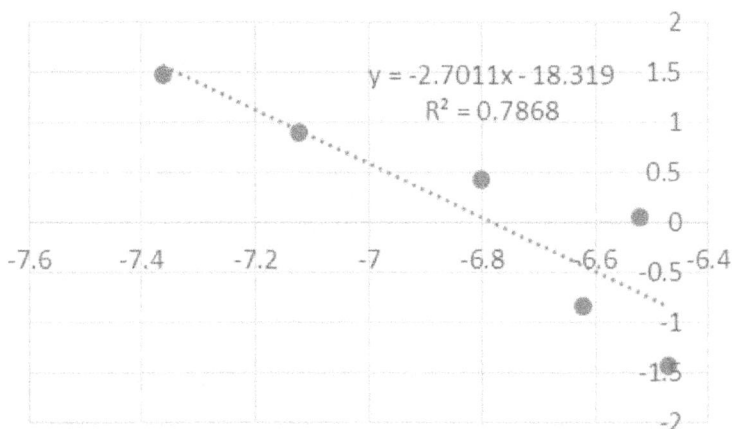

Figure 10.
Linear correlation between docking score and bioactivity ($-\log IC_{50}$). Docking was performed with the standard settings of MOE.

In an attempt to attain a quantitative measure of ligand-binding affinity, the docking scores of the compounds were graphed against observed potencies (**Figure 10**). Potencies had been obtained in cell viability assays and the underlying assumption was that ligand binding to the receptor constituted the critical step that would lead to cell toxicity and therefore would correlate with bioactivity. **Figure 10** shows a reasonable correlation between the two quantities with a squared correlation coefficient of 0.79. This data is consistent with the proposed binding mode of AhR ligands, which relies predominately on hydrophobic but also on additional π-π interactions.

4. Molecular dynamics simulations

We complemented our docking-based analysis by MD simulations, whose purpose was twofold. First, we wanted to ensure the stability of a docked pose by monitoring its behavior in a time-resolved system. Second, MD simulations can reveal the role of explicit solvent molecules, something that cannot be accounted for by docking. We selected compound 7 as a representative and subjected it to a simulation time of 100 ns, using the CHARMM36m force field for the protein [22] and the CHARMM general force field for the ligand [23]. The parameters for water were taken from the CHARMM-modified TIP3P water model [24–26] to match those used for the solute. The initial structure of the protein-ligand complex was obtained from docking experiments, and the simulation was performed with the software NAMD [27].

As shown in **Figure 11**, the differences between the poses before and after 100 ns of simulation time were minor. The overall position of the ligand did not change significantly and the only notable difference related to a slight rotation around the central axis of the molecule which placed the nitrile group in a somewhat different environment.

Interestingly, analysis of the MD simulation data revealed the presence of several water molecules in close proximity to the ligand. This observation was somewhat unexpected; while polar water molecules have been found in predominately hydrophobic cores of proteins, it is a rare occurrence [28, 29]. Residues exposed to water molecules included Leu315, Thr289, His 291, Gln383, Ser365, and His 337. In some cases, the solvent molecules formed bridged hydrogen bonds between the nitrile group and the ligand. The latter could explain the abovementioned slight twist of the nitrile group into a more favorable position.

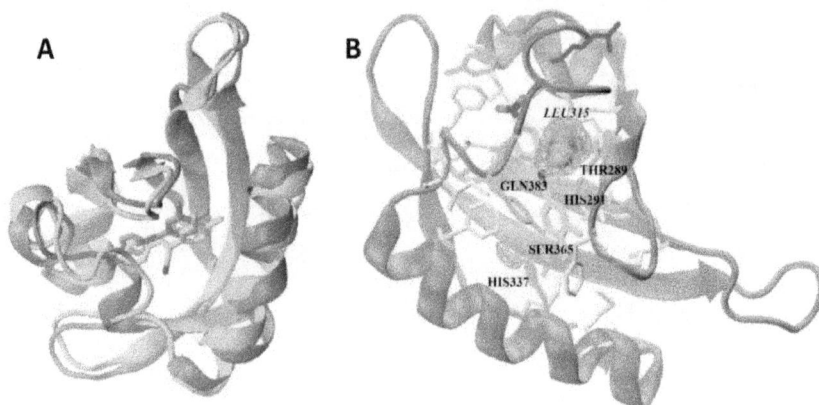

Figure 11.
MD simulations. (A) Ligand/AhR complex before (gray) and after (blue) 100 ns of simulation time. (B) Density of water molecules in the binding site as highlighted by orange grids. Residues are colored according to their polarity (pink: nonpolar; green: polar uncharged).

5. Conclusions

Using the AhR and substituted phenylacrylonitriles as an example, we demonstrated the usefulness of a number of computational tools for the study of ligand/receptor interactions. Homology modeling gave access to the structure of a protein domain that has not yet been solved by X-ray crystallography. The most probable binding site was identified, allowing for the docking of ligands, along with a good estimate of their affinities. The identification of this docking site was consistent with subsequent compound design and biological data obtained [10]. MD simulations validated the stability of docked poses and illustrated the role of solvent molecules in the binding pocket. The value of the described techniques lies in their ability to rapidly evaluate the potential of a new ligand in silico before spending precious time and resource on its synthesis and experimental evaluation.

Acknowledgements

JR Baker is the grateful recipient of an Australian Government Research Training Program (RTP) scholarship. This work was conducted in part under the auspices of a Fulbright Fellowship awarded to S Paula.

Conflict of interest

The authors declare no conflicts of interest.

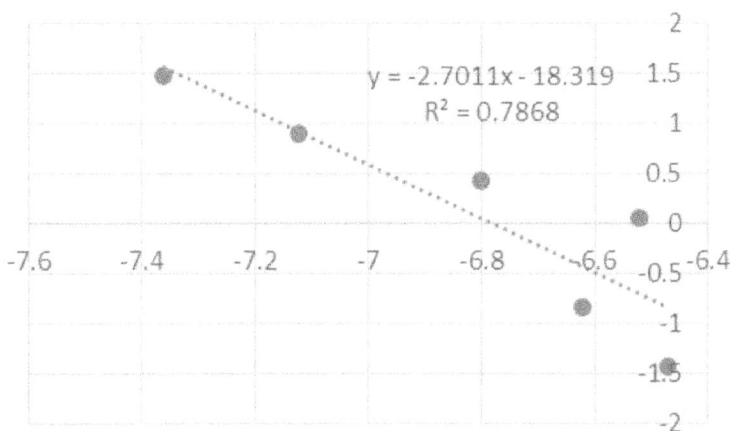

$$y = -2.7011x - 18.319$$
$$R^2 = 0.7868$$

Figure 10.
Linear correlation between docking score and bioactivity ($-\log IC_{50}$). Docking was performed with the standard settings of MOE.

In an attempt to attain a quantitative measure of ligand-binding affinity, the docking scores of the compounds were graphed against observed potencies (**Figure 10**). Potencies had been obtained in cell viability assays and the underlying assumption was that ligand binding to the receptor constituted the critical step that would lead to cell toxicity and therefore would correlate with bioactivity. **Figure 10** shows a reasonable correlation between the two quantities with a squared correlation coefficient of 0.79. This data is consistent with the proposed binding mode of AhR ligands, which relies predominately on hydrophobic but also on additional π-π interactions.

4. Molecular dynamics simulations

We complemented our docking-based analysis by MD simulations, whose purpose was twofold. First, we wanted to ensure the stability of a docked pose by monitoring its behavior in a time-resolved system. Second, MD simulations can reveal the role of explicit solvent molecules, something that cannot be accounted for by docking. We selected compound 7 as a representative and subjected it to a simulation time of 100 ns, using the CHARMM36m force field for the protein [22] and the CHARMM general force field for the ligand [23]. The parameters for water were taken from the CHARMM-modified TIP3P water model [24–26] to match those used for the solute. The initial structure of the protein-ligand complex was obtained from docking experiments, and the simulation was performed with the software NAMD [27].

As shown in **Figure 11**, the differences between the poses before and after 100 ns of simulation time were minor. The overall position of the ligand did not change significantly and the only notable difference related to a slight rotation around the central axis of the molecule which placed the nitrile group in a somewhat different environment.

Interestingly, analysis of the MD simulation data revealed the presence of several water molecules in close proximity to the ligand. This observation was somewhat unexpected; while polar water molecules have been found in predominately hydrophobic cores of proteins, it is a rare occurrence [28, 29]. Residues exposed to water molecules included Leu315, Thr289, His 291, Gln383, Ser365, and His 337. In some cases, the solvent molecules formed bridged hydrogen bonds between the nitrile group and the ligand. The latter could explain the abovementioned slight twist of the nitrile group into a more favorable position.

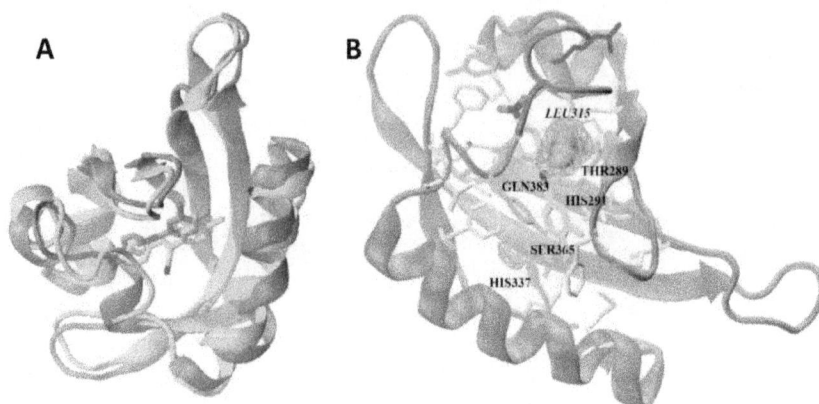

Figure 11.
MD simulations. (A) Ligand/AhR complex before (gray) and after (blue) 100 ns of simulation time. (B) Density of water molecules in the binding site as highlighted by orange grids. Residues are colored according to their polarity (pink: nonpolar; green: polar uncharged).

5. Conclusions

Using the AhR and substituted phenylacrylonitriles as an example, we demonstrated the usefulness of a number of computational tools for the study of ligand/receptor interactions. Homology modeling gave access to the structure of a protein domain that has not yet been solved by X-ray crystallography. The most probable binding site was identified, allowing for the docking of ligands, along with a good estimate of their affinities. The identification of this docking site was consistent with subsequent compound design and biological data obtained [10]. MD simulations validated the stability of docked poses and illustrated the role of solvent molecules in the binding pocket. The value of the described techniques lies in their ability to rapidly evaluate the potential of a new ligand in silico before spending precious time and resource on its synthesis and experimental evaluation.

Acknowledgements

JR Baker is the grateful recipient of an Australian Government Research Training Program (RTP) scholarship. This work was conducted in part under the auspices of a Fulbright Fellowship awarded to S Paula.

Conflict of interest

The authors declare no conflicts of interest.

Author details

Stefan Paula[1*], Jennifer R. Baker[2], Xiao Zhu[3] and Adam McCluskey[2]

1 Department of Chemistry, Purdue University, West Lafayette, Indiana, USA

2 Centre for Chemical Biology, Chemistry, School of Environmental Life Science, The University of Newcastle, Callaghan, New South Wales, Australia

3 Research Computing, Information Technology at Purdue (ITaP), Purdue University, West Lafayette, IN, USA

*Address all correspondence to: paulas@purdue.edu

IntechOpen

References

[1] Powell JB, Goode GD, Eltom SE. The aryl hydrocarbon receptor: A target for breast cancer therapy. Journal of Cancer Therapy. 2014;**4**(7):1177-1186. DOI: 10.4236/jct.2013.47137

[2] Haarmann-Stemmann T, Bothe H, Abel J. Growth factors, cytokines and their receptors as downstream targets of the arylhydrocarbon receptor (AhR) signaling pathways. Biochemical Pharmacology. 2009;77(4):508-520. DOI: 10.1016/j.bcp.2008.09.013

[3] Kung T, Murphy KA, White LA. The arylhydrocarbon receptor (AhR) pathway as a regulatory pathway for cell adhesion and matrix metabolism. Biochemical Pharmacology. 2009;77(4):536-546. DOI: 10.1016/j.bcp.2008.09.031

[4] Hanieh H, Mohafez O, Hairul-Islam VI, Alzahrani A, Bani Ismail M, Thirugnanasambantham K. Novel aryl hydrocarbon receptor agonist suppresses migration and invasion of breast cancer cells. PLoS One. 2016;4(1):1-16. DOI: 10.1371/journal.pone.0167650

[5] Bradshaw TD, Bell DR. Relevance of the aryl hydrocarbon receptor (AhR) for clinical toxicology. Clinical Toxicology. 2009;47(7):632-642. DOI: 10.1080/15563650903140423

[6] Mandal PK. Dioxin: A review of its environmental effects and its aryl hydrocarbon receptor biology. Journal of Comparative Physiology B: Biochemical, Systemic, and Environmental Physiology. 2005;175(4):221-230. DOI: 10.1007/s00360-005-0483-3

[7] Stockinger B, Meglio P, D, Gialitakis M, Duarte JH. The aryl hydrocarbon receptor: Multitasking in the immune system. Annual Review of Immunology. 2014;32(1):403-432. DOI: 10.1146/annurev-immunol-032713-120245

[8] Brantley E, Callero MA, Berardi DE, Campbell P, Rowland L, Zylstra D, et al. AhR ligand aminoflavone inhibits A6-integrin expression and breast cancer sphere-initiating capacity. Cancer Letters. 2016;376(1):53-61. DOI: 10.1016/j.canlet.2016.03.025

[9] Tarleton M, Gilbert J, Robertson MJ, McCluskey A, Sakoff JA. Library synthesis and cytotoxicity of a family of 2-phenylacrylonitriles and discovery of an estrogen dependent breast cancer lead compound. MedChemComm. 2011;2(1):31-37. DOI: 10.1039/c0md00147c

[10] Baker JR, Gilbert J, Paula S, Zhu X, Sakoff JA, McCluskey A. Dichlorophenylacrylonitriles as AhR ligands that display selective breast cancer cytotoxicity in vitro. ChemMedChem. 2018;13:1447-1458. DOI: 10.1002/cmdc.201800256

[11] Akama T, Shida Y, Sugaya T, Ishida H, Gomi K, Kasai M. Novel 5-aminoflavone derivatives as specific antitumor agents in breast cancer. Journal of Medicinal Chemistry. 1996;39(18):3461-3469. DOI: 10.1021/jm950938g

[12] Shi D, Bradshaw TD, Wrigley S, Mccall CJ, Lelieveld P, Fichtner I, et al. Antitumour benzothiazoles. 3. Synthesis of 2-(4-aminophenyl)benzothiazoles and evaluation of their activities against breast cancer cell lines in vitro and in vivo. Journal of Medicinal Chemistry. 1996;39(17):3375-3384. DOI: 10.1109/ICCCN.2012.6289316

[13] Gilbert J, De Iuliis GN, Tarleton M, McCluskey A, Sakoff J. (Z)-2-(3,4-dichlorophenyl)-3-(1H-pyrrol-2-yl) acrylonitrile exhibits selective anti-tumour activity in breast cancer cell lines via the aryl hydrocarbon receptor pathway. Molecular Pharmacology. 2018;93(2):168-177. DOI: 10.1124/mol.117.109827

[14] Huang N, Chelliah Y, Shan Y, Taylor CA, Yoo S-H, Partch C, et al. Crystal structure of the heterodimeric CLOCK:BMAL1 transcriptional activator complex. Science. 2012;**337**(6091): 189-194. DOI: 10.1126/science.1222804

[15] King HA, Hoelz A, Crane BR, Young MW. Structure of an enclosed dimer formed by the *Drosophila* period protein. Journal of Molecular Biology. 2011;**413**(3):561-572. DOI: 10.1016/j. jmb.2011.08.048

[16] Correia C, Wasielewski E, Prendergast F, Mer G. Structure of human circadian clock protein BMAL2 C-terminal PAS domain. Available from: www.rcsb.org/structure/2KDK [Accessed: October 01/2019]. DOI: 10.2210/PDB2KDK/PDB

[17] Sliwoski G, Kothiwale S, Meiler J, Lowe EW. Computational methods in drug discovery. Pharmacological Reviews. 2014;**66**(1):334-395. DOI: 10.1124/pr.112.007336

[18] Arnold K, Bordoli L, Kopp J, Schwede T. The SWISS-MODEL workspace: A web-based environment for protein structure homology modelling. Bioinformatics. 2006;**22**(2):195-201. DOI: 10.1093/bioinformatics/bti770

[19] Wu D, Su X, Potluri N, Kim Y, Rastinejad F. NPAS1-ARNT and NPAS3-ARNT crystal structures implicate the bHLH-PAS as multi-ligand binding transcription factors. eLife. 2016;**5**(e18790):1-15. DOI: 10.7554/eLife.18790

[20] Scheuermann TH, Tomchick DR, Machius M, Guo Y, Bruick RK, Gardner KH. Artificial ligand binding within the HIF2α PAS-B domain of the HIF2 transcription factor. PNAS. 2009;**106**(2):450-455. DOI: 10.1073/pnas.0808092106

[21] Key J, Scheuermann TH, Anderson PC, Daggett V, Gardner KH. Principles of ligand binding within a completely buried cavity in HIF2α PAS-B. Journal of the American Chemical Society. 2009;**131**(48):17647-17654. DOI: 10.1021/ja9073062

[22] Huang J, Rauscher S, Nawrocki G, Ran T, Feig M, de Groot BL, et al. CHARMM36m: An improved force field for folded and intrinsically disordered proteins. Nature Methods. 2017;**14**(1):71-73. DOI: 10.1038/nmeth.4067

[23] Vanommeslaeghe K, Hatcher E, Acharya C, Kundu S, Zhong S, Shim J, et al. CHARMM general force field: A force field for drug-like molecules compatible with the CHARMM all-atom additive biological force fields. Journal of Computational Chemistry. 2010;**31**(4):671-690. DOI: 10.1002/jcc.21367

[24] Jorgensen WL, Chandrasekhar J, Madura JD, Impey RW, Klein ML. Comparison of simple potential functions for simulating liquid water. The Journal of Chemical Physics. 1983;**79**(2):926-935. DOI: 10.1063/1.445869

[25] Durell SR, Brooks BR, Ben-Naim A. Solvent-induced forces between two hydrophilic groups. The Journal of Physical Chemistry. 1994;**98**(8): 2198-2202. DOI: 10.1021/j100059a038

[26] Neria E, Fischer S, Karplus M. Simulation of activation free energies in molecular systems. The Journal of Chemical Physics. 1996;**105**(5): 1902-1921. DOI: 10.1063/1.472061

[27] Phillips JC, Braun R, Wang W, Gumbart J, Tajkhorshid E, Villa E, et al. Scalable molecular dynamics with NAMD. Journal of Computational Chemistry. 2005;**26**:1781-1802. DOI: 10.1002/jcc.20289

[28] Levy Y, Onuchic J. Water and proteins: A love-hate relationship. PNAS. 2004;**101**(10):3325-3326. DOI: 10.1073/pnas.0400157101

[29] Adamek DH, Guerrero L, Blaber M, Caspar DLD. Structural and energetic consequences of mutations in a solvated hydrophobic cavity. Journal of Molecular Biology. 2005;**346**(1):307-318. DOI: 10.1016/j.jmb.2004.11.046

Chapter 3

In Silico Drug Design and Molecular Docking Studies of Some Quinolone Compound

Lucia Pintilie and Amalia Stefaniu

Abstract

Quinolones are an important class of heterocyclic compounds that possess interesting biological activities like antimicrobial, antitubercular, and antitumor. The objective of this study is to evaluate in *silico* the antitumoral and antimycobacterial activity of some quinolone derivatives by using CLC Drug Discovery Workbench Software. Docking studies were carried out for all ligands, and the docking scores were compared with the scores of standard drugs, topotecan and levofloxacin. The docking studies have been carried out to predict the most possible type of interaction, the binding affinities, and the orientations of the docked ligands at the active site of the target protein.

Keywords: molecular docking, quinolones, antimicrobial activity, antitumoral activity, antimycobacterial activity

1. Introduction

In medical practice, many quinolone derivatives with antimicrobial activity are used; some of these being considered by pharmacists as the primary drugs in human and veterinary anti-infectious therapy. Quinolones have a broad spectrum and a strong antibacterial activity [1, 2]. They are characterized by pharmacokinetics that allows their use in all localized infections. Recently, pharmacological studies have shown that quinolones also possess other biological activities: antitumor activity [3–6], antimycobaterial activity [7], antiviral activity on herpes virus, inhibiting neurovegetative diseases and ischemic infections, and food product storage (due to bactericidal properties). First antitumoral quinolone is Voreloxin: (+)-1,4-dihydro-7-(3S4S)-3-hydroxy-4-amino-1-pyrrolidinyl-4-oxo-1-(2-thiazolyl)-1.8-naphthyridine-3-carboxylic acid (**Figure 1**) [3]. Some quinolone derivatives (e.g., Moxifloxacin: 1-cyclopropyl-6-fluoro-7-((4aS,7aS)-hexahydro-1H-pyrrolo[3,4-b]pyridin-6(2H)-yl)-8-methoxy-4-oxo-1,4-dihydroquinoline-3-carboxylic acid-**Figure 2**) show activity against *Mycobacterium tuberculosis,* and these compounds are the first new antimycobacterial drugs to be available since the discovery of rifampin [8].

Lascufloxacin (AM-1977) (**Figure 3**) [9, 10] is a new 8-methoxy fluoroquinolone antibacterial agent with unique pharmacophores at the first and seventh positions of the quinolone rings. The oral and parenteral formulations have been developed for the treatment of community-acquired pneumonia and other respiratory tract infections in Japan. Lascufloxacin shows *in vitro* activity against various respiratory

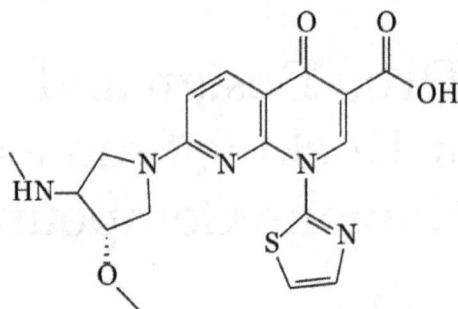

Figure 1.
Voreloxin.

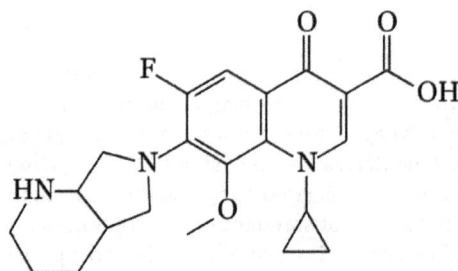

Figure 2.
Moxifloxacin.

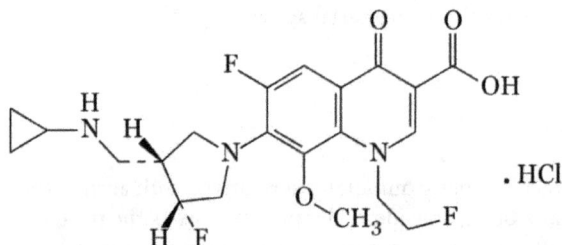

Figure 3.
Lascufloxacin.

pathogens, such as *Staphylococcus aureus*, *Streptococcus pneumoniae*, *Moraxella catarrhalis*, *Haemophilus influenzae*, and *Mycoplasma pneumoniae*.

Quinolones, considered to be "privileged building blocks," are obtained through simple and flexible synthesis methods and allow design and development of large libraries of bioactive molecules. A 2011 study on 21 antibiotics launched since 2000 has highlighted that the discovery and development of new antibiotics obtained through chemical synthesis is still topical. Of the nine antibiotics obtained by chemical synthesis, launched between 2000 and 2011, eight antibiotics belong to the class of fluoroquinolones [11]. New drugs introduced into medical therapies each year are privileged structures for specific biological targets. These new chemical entities provide a perspective on molecular recognition, serving as a basis for designing future new drugs. In 2016, 19 chemically synthesized drugs were approved [12], with the two drugs having the quinolone structure: nemonoxacin (**Figure 4**) and zabofloxacin (**Figure 5**).

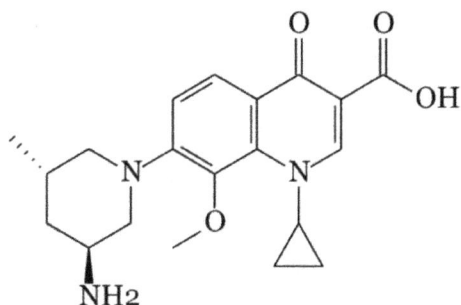

Figure 4.
Nemonoxacin (Taigexyn).

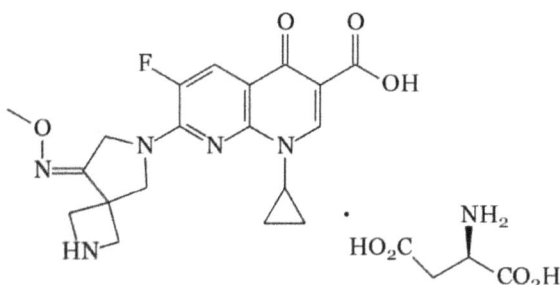

Figure 5.
Zaboflaxacin D-aspartate.

The objective of this study is to evaluate *"in silico"* antitumoral and antimyco-bacterial activities of some quinolone derivatives by using CLC Drug Discovery Workbench Software [13]. Docking studies were conducted for all ligands, and the docking scores were compared with the scores of standard drugs, topotecan and levofloxacin.

2. Materials and methods

2.1 Structure and the synthesis pathway of the quinolone derivatives

In previous papers, we presented the synthesis of quinolone derivatives with antimicrobial activity [1, 2]. The results have revealed that the compounds represented in **Figure 6** have showed weak antibacterial activities against the tested strains. For this reason, we have initiated *in silico* drug design and molecular docking studies to predict anticancer and antitubercular activities targeting DNA-topoisomerase I and topoisomerase IV from *Klebsiella pneumoniae*, respectively.

We have performed molecular docking studies to see how the nature of sub-stituents on the quinolone ring influences the anticancer and antitubercular activi-ties targeting human DNA topoisomerase I and topoisomerase IV from *Klebsiella pneumoniae*, respectively. The studies have been realized with CLC Drug Discovery Workbench Software [13] in order to achieve accurate predictions on optimized conformations for both the quinolones (as ligands) and their target receptor pro-teins to form stable complexes.

The quinolone compounds have been synthesized by Gould-Jacobs cyclization process (**Figure 7**). Appropriate unsubstituted aniline (**1**) is reacted with diethyl

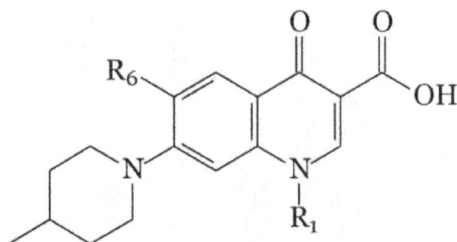

Figure 6.
General structure of the investigated quinolone compounds, where R_1 = allyl, isopropyl, benzyl, p-nitro-phenyl, p-amino-phenyl and R_6 = F, Cl, H, CH$_3$.

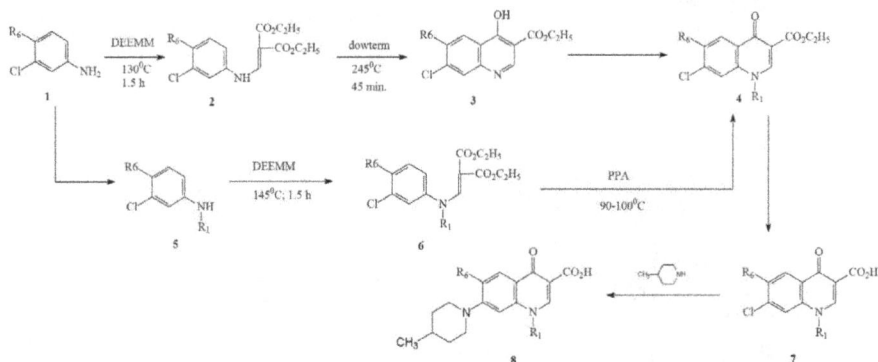

Figure 7.
The synthesis of the quinolone compound using Gould-Jacobs cyclization process.

ethoxymethylenemalonate (DEEMM) to produce the anilinomethylene malonate derivatives (**2**). A subsequent thermal process induces Gould-Jacobs cyclization to afford the corresponding 4-hydroxy-quinoline-3-carboxylate ethyl ester (**3**). The following operation is the alkylation/arylation of the quinolone compound (**4**), which is usually accomplished by reaction with allyl chloride, benzyl chloride, or *para* fluoronitrobenzene to produce the qinolone-3-carboxylate ester (**4**) (R_1 = allyl, benzyl, *para* nitrophenyl) [14–16, 19, 20]. The qinolone-3-carboxylate ester (**4**) (R_1 = *iso*propyl) was obtained by the reaction of the corresponding monosubstituted aniline (**5**) (R_1 = *iso*propyl) (the aniline (**5**) was obtained by reductive amination of acetone with sodium borohydride-acetic acid [14–16, 19] or triacetoxyborohydride [17, 18]) with DEEMM. A strong acid (such as polyphosphoric acid) is often needed to induce cyclization directly resulting in the formation of N-*iso*propyl-4-oxo-quinolone-3-carboxylate ester (**4**) (R_1 = *iso*propyl).

The final manipulation is the basic or acid hydrolysis that cleave the ester generating the biologically active free carboxylic acid (**7**) (R_1 = allyl, *iso*propyl, benzyl, *para* nitrophenyl). The displacement of 7-chloro group from the biologically active free carboxylic acid (**7**) with 4-methyl-piperidine yielded the compound (**8**) (R_1 = allyl, benzyl, *iso*propyl, *para* nitrophenyl) (**Table 1**). The quinolone compounds (**8**) (R_1 = *para* amino phenyl) (**Table 1**) have been synthesized by a common reduction of nitro group using sodium dithionite [20].

2.2 Ligand preparation

To achieve the docking studies, the quinolone derivatives (ligands) must be prepared to be imported in the molecular docking project. The ligands (**Table 1**)

Quinolone derivatives	2D structures	3D optimized structures
PQ4:1-allyl-6-fluoro-7-(4-methyl-piperidin-1-yl)-1,4-dihydro-4-oxo-quinolin-3-carboxylic acid [14] E: −1171.69431 au		
6ClPQ4:1-allyl-6-chloro-7-(4-methyl-piperidin-1-yl)-1,4-dihydro-4-oxo-quinolin-3-carboxylic acid [19] E: −1532.05076 au		
HPQ4:1-allyl-7-(4-methyl-piperidin-1-yl)-1,4-dihydro-4-oxo-quinolin-3-carboxylic acid [15] E: −1072.46696 au		
6MePQ4:1-allyl-6-methyl-7-(4-methyl-piperidin-1-yl)-1,4-dihydro-4-oxo-quinolin-3-carboxylic acid [16] E: −1111.77842 au		
PQ12:1-*iso*propyl-6-fluoro-7-(4-methyl-piperidin-1-yl)-1,4-dihydro-4-oxo-quinolin-3-carboxylic acid [14] E: −1172.93189 au		
6ClPQ12:1-*iso*propyl-6-chloro-7-(4-methyl-piperidin-1-yl)-1,4-dihydro-4-oxo-quinolin-3-carboxylic acid [19] E: −1533.28880 au		
HPQ12:1-*iso*propyl-7-(4-methyl-piperidin-1-yl)-1,4-dihydro-4-oxo-quinolin-3-carboxylic acid [15] E: −1073.70428 au		
6MePQ12:1-*iso*propyl-6-methyl-7-(4-methyl-piperidin-1-yl)-1,4-dihydro-4-oxo-quinolin-3-carboxylic acid [16] E: −1113.01581 au		
PQ11:1-benzyl-6-fluoro-7-(4-methyl-piperidin-1-yl)-1,4-dihydro-4-oxo-quinolin-3-carboxylic acid [14] E: −1325.35417 au		

Quinolone derivatives	2D structures	3D optimized structures
6ClPQ11:1-benzyl-6-chloro-7-(4-methyl-piperidin-1-yl)-1,4-dihydro-4-oxo-quinolin-3-carboxylic acid [19] E: −1685.71018 au		
HPQ11:1-benzyl-7-(4-methyl-piperidin-1-yl)-1,4-dihydro-4-oxo-quinolin-3-carboxylic acid [15] E: −1226.12649 au		
6MePQ11:1-benzyl-6-methyl-7-(4-methyl-piperidin-1-yl)-1,4-dihydro-4-oxo-quinolin-3-carboxylic acid [16] E: −1265.46016 au		
PQ13:1-(*p*-nitro-phenyl)-6-fluoro-7-(4-methyl-piperidin-1-yl)-1,4-dihydro-4-oxo-quinolin-3-carboxylic acid [20] E: −1490.53723 au		
6ClPQ13:1-(*p*-nitro-phenyl)-6-chloro-7-(4-methyl-piperidin-1-yl)-1,4-dihydro-4-oxo-quinolin-3-carboxylic acid [20] E: −1850.89287 au		
HPQ13:1-(*p*-nitro-phenyl)-7-(4-methyl-piperidin-1-yl)-1,4-dihydro-4-oxo-quinolin-3-carboxylic acid E: −1391.31010 au		
6MePQ13:1-(*p*-nitro-phenyl)-6-methyl-7-(4-methyl-piperidin-1-yl)-1,4-dihydro-4-oxo-quinolin-3-carboxylic acid [20] E: −430.62213 au		
APQ13:1-(*p*-amino-phenyl)-6-fluoro-7-(4-methyl-piperidin-1-yl)-1,4-dihydro-4-oxo-quinolin-3-carboxylic acid [20] E: −1341.39572 au		

Quinolone derivatives	2D structures	3D optimized structures
A6ClPQ13: 1-(*p*-amino-phenyl)-6-chloro-7-(4-methyl-piperidin-1-yl)-1,4-dihydro-4-oxo-quinolin-3-carboxylic acid E: −1701.75238 au		
AHPQ13:1-(*p*-amino-phenyl)-7-(4-methyl-piperidin-1-yl)-1,4-dihydro-4-oxo-quinolin-3-carboxylic acid E: −1242.16807 au		
A6MePQ13:1-(*p*-amino-phenyl)-6-methyl-7-(4-methyl-piperidin-1-yl)-1,4-dihydro-4-oxo-quinolin-3-carboxylic acid [20] E: −1281.47987 au		

E = energy and au = atomic units.

Table 1.
The 2D and 3D structures of the quinolone compounds.

have been prepared using SPARTAN'14 software package [21] according to the protocol described in our previous work [22]. The DFT/B3LYP/6-31 G* level of basis set has been used for the computation of molecular structure, vibrational frequencies, and energies of optimized structures.

Some chemical properties, highest occupied molecular orbital (HOMO) and lowest unoccupied molecular orbital (LUMO) energy values, HOMO and LUMO orbital coefficient distribution, molecular dipole moment, polar surface area (PSA) (a descriptor that has been shown to correlate well with passive molecular transport through membranes, therefore, allows the prediction of transport properties of the drugs), the ovality, polarizability (useful to predict the interactions between non-polar atoms or groups and other electrically charged species, such as ions and polar molecules having a strong dipole moment), and the octanol water partition coefficient (log P) have been calculated (**Table 2**).

2.3 Docking studies

The docking protocol was performed according to the CLC Drug Discovery Workbench Software and was described in a previous paper [22]. The docking scores and hydrogen bonds formed with the amino acids from group interaction atoms were used to predict the binding modes, the binding affinities, and the orientation of the docked quinolone derivatives in the active site of the target proteins.

2.3.1 Docking evaluation against human DNA topoisomerase

Docking studies have been carried out in order to achieve accurate predictions on the optimized conformations for both the quinolone derivatives (as ligands) and

Compounds	Molecular properties									
	Dipole moment (Debye)	E HOMO (eV)	E LUMO (eV)	HOMO-LUMO GAP	Polarizability (10^{-30} m³)	PSA (Å²)	Ovality	Log P	HBA count	HBD count
PQ4	11.42	-5.88	-1.62	4.28	68.31	44.205	1.51	2.92	1	4
6ClPQ4	9.50	-6.24	-1.91	4.33	69.10	44.864	1.52	3.32	1	4
HPQ4	11.77	-5.85	-1.47	4.38	67.89	44.618	1.50	2.76	1	4
6MePQ4	11.65	-5.77	-1.43	4.34	69.36	44.396	1.51	3.35	1	4
PQ11	11.37	-5.88	-1.62	4.26	72.46	44.195	1.55	4.44	1	4
6ClPQ11	9.67	-6.18	-1.89	4.29	73.27	44.610	1.57	4.84	1	4
HPQ11	11.82	-5.82	-1.46	4.36	72.05	44.426	1.54	4.29	1	4
6MePQ11	11.78	-5.74	-1.40	4.34	73.50	44.271	1.55	3.38	1	4
PQ12	11.19	-5.94	-1.62	4.32	68.57	44.362	1.51	3.37	1	4
6ClPQ12	9.55	-6.18	-1.86	4.32	69.36	44.844	1.52	3.77	1	4
HPQ12	11.68	-5.88	-1.44	4.44	68.15	44.658	1.50	3.21	1	4
6MePQ12	11.16	-5.78	-1.38	4.40	69.64	44.246	1.50	3.70	1	4
PQ13	9.37	-6.03	-3.08	2.95	73.03	82.971	1.57	0.10	1	7
6ClPQ13	6.99	-6.37	-3.13	3.24	73.76	83.732	1.58	0.50	1	7
HPQ13	10.10	-6.06	-3.01	3.05	72.60	83.520	1.56	-0.06	1	7
6MePQ13	9.78	-5.98	-3.01	2.97	74.07	83.336	1.57	0.43	1	7
APQ13	13.57	-5.81	-1.49	4.32	71.82	61.120	1.56	2.75	2	5
6ClAPQ13	12.11	-6.11	-1.74	4.37	72.62	69.491	1.58	3.15	2	5
HAPQ13	13.91	-5.76	-1.32	4.44	71.41	69.419	1.55	2.59	2	5

Table 2.
Molecular properties for CPK model computations for quinolone compounds.

protein target to form a stable complex. All of the investigated compounds have been docked on the crystal structure of human DNA topoisomerase I (PDB ID: 1K4T) [23]. Binding site and docking pose of the co-crystallized topotecan (TTC), interacting with amino acid residues of the active site, are shown in **Figure 8a**. The TTC was taken as reference ligand to compare the docking results of quinolone derivatives. The docking score, the interacting group, and hydrogen bonds formed with the group interaction atoms of the corresponding amino acids are shown in **Table 3**. Interactions of quinolone derivatives PQ11 (score: −63.31 and RMSD: 0.12), 6ClPQ11 (score: −62.95 and RMSD: 0.08), HPQ11 (score: −62.77 and RMSD: 0.06), 6MePQ11(score: −62.48 and RMSD: 0.01), and 6MePQ13 (score: −61.22 and RMSD: 0.04) showed better docking score than that of co-crystalized TTC (score: −59.15 and RMSD: 0.14) as shown in **Figures 8b–11a**. The most active compound, 6ClPQ11, was predicted to have a significant docking score (−63.31) and forms one hydrogen bond with GLU 418 (bond length − 2.961 Å) (**Figure 9a**). Docking poses of all quinolone derivatives in the ligand binding site of human DNA topoisomerase I are shown in **Figure 11b**.

2.3.2 Docking evaluation against topoisomerase IV from Klebsiella pneumoniae

Docking studies have been carried out in order to obtain optimized docking conformations of the investigated quinolone derivatives on the crystal structure of topoisomerase IV (PDB ID: 5EIX) from *Klebsiella pneumoniae* [24]. The binding site and docking pose of the co-crystallized levofloxacin (LFX) ligand, interacting with amino acid residues of the ligand binding site of topoisomerase IV from *Klebsiella pneumoniae*, are shown in **Figure 12a**. The levofloxacin was taken as reference ligand to compare the docking results of quinolone derivatives. The docking score, the interacting group, and hydrogen bonds formed with the group interaction atoms of the corresponding amino acids are shown in **Table 4**. Interactions of quinolone derivatives PQ4 (score: −43.98 and RMSD: 0.05), 6ClPQ4 (score: −41.12 and RMSD: 0.25), PQ11 (score: −48.32 and RMSD: 0.10), HPQ11 (score: 49.57 and RMSD: 0.11), PQ12 (score: −42.76 and RMSD: 0.18), and APQ13 (score: −42.96 and RMSD: 0.32) showed better docking score than that of co-crystalized LFX (score: 37.26 and RMSD: 0.02) as shown in **Figures 12b–15a**. The most active compound,

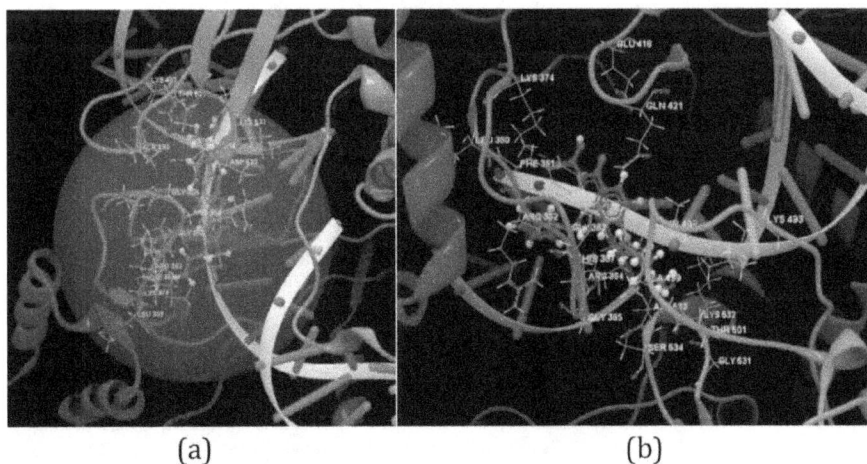

(a) (b)

Figure 8.
(a) Binding site and docking pose of the co-crystallized TTC ligand interacting with the amino acid residues of the ligand binding site of human DNA topoisomerase I. (b) Docking pose of the PQ11 ligand interacting with the amino acid residues of the ligand binding site of human DNA topoisomerase I.

Ligand	Score/ RMSD (Å)	Group interaction/hydrogen bond	Bond length (Å)
TTC D-990	−59.15/ 0.14	LYS 493, THR 501, LYS 532, GLY 531, ALA 499, THR 498, SER 534, ASP 533, GLY 365, ARG 364, HIS 367, GLY 363, ARG 362, PHE 361, LYS 374, and LEU 360	
		O sp^3 from TTC– N sp^2 from ASP 533	3.065
		O sp^3 from TTC– O sp^3 from THR 501	3.166
		N sp^2 from TTC– N sp^2 from ARG 364	3.353
		O sp^3 from TTC– O sp^2 from GLY 363	3.112
		O sp^3 from TTC– N sp^2 from GLY 363	3.038
PQ4	−55.35/ 0.07	GLU 418, GLN 421, LYS 374, THR 498, PHE 361, GLY 363, HIS 367, ARG 364, ARG 362, GLY 365, SER 534, ASP 533, ALA 499, GLY 531, THR 501, ASP 500, and LYS 532	
		O sp^3 from CO$_2$H(OH)-N sp^3 from LYS 374	3.124
6ClPQ4	−55.81/ 0.12	LYS 425, TRP 416, ARG 364, GLY 363, ILE 377, ARG 362, PHE 361, LYS 374, ARG 375, LEU 360, MET 263, ILE 420, ASN 419, GLN 421, and GLU 418	
		O sp^3 from CO$_2$H(CO)-N sp^2 from ARG 364	3.056
		O sp^3 from CO$_2$H (OH)-O sp^2 from GLY 363	2.808
		O sp^2 from CO-N sp^2 from ARG 364	3.009
HPQ4	−56.08/ 0.10	ARG 364, LYS 425, GLY 363, ARG 362, GLN 421, GLU 418, PHE 361, ILE 420, ASN 118, LYS 374, ARG 375, ILE 377, LEU 360, and MET 263	
		O sp^3 from CO$_2$H(CO)-N sp^2 from ARG 364	2.782
		O sp^2 from CO-N sp^2 from ARG 364	2.887
6MePQ4	−55.52/ 0.10	GLU 418, GLN 421, LYS 374, THR 498, PHE 361, GLY 363, HIS 367, ARG 364, ARG 362, GLY 365, SER 534, ASP 533, ALA 499, GLY 531, THR 501, and LYS 532	
		O sp^3 from CO$_2$H (OH)-N sp^3 from LYS 374	3.040
PQ11	−62.95/ 0.08	GLU 418, GLN 421, LYS 374, LEU 360, THR 498, PHE 361, GLY 363, HIS 367, ARG 364, ARG 362, LYS 493, GLY 365, SER 534, ASP 533, ALA 499, GLY 531, THR 501, and LYS 532	
		O sp^3 from CO$_2$H (OH)-N sp^3 from LYS 374	3.214
6ClPQ11	−63.31/ 0.12	SER 423, LYS 425, GLN 421, GLU 418, ILE 420, LYS 374, LYS 493, THR 498, LYS 532, GLY 531, THR 501, ASP 533, ALA 499, SER 534, ARG 364, GLY 365, GLY 363, HIS 367, ARG 362, PHE 361, and LEU 360	
		O sp^3 from CO$_2$H(OH)-O sp^2 from GLU 418	2.961
HPQ11	−62.77/ 0.06	SER 423, LYS 425, GLN 421, GLU 418, ILE 420, LYS 374, LYS 493, THR 498, LYS 532, GLY 531, THR 501, ASP 533, ALA 499, SER 534, ARG 364, GLY 365, GLY 363, HIS 367, ARG 362, PHE 361, and LEU 360	
		O sp^2 from CO$_2$H(OH)-O sp^2 from ASP 533	3.144
		O sp^3 from CO$_2$H(CO)-N sp^2 from ARG 364	3.111
		O sp^3 from CO$_2$H(CO)-N sp^2 from ARG 364	2.748
6MePQ11	−62.48/ 0.01	GLU 418, GLN 421, LYS 374, THR 498, PHE 361, GLY 363, HIS 367, ARG 364, ARG 362, LYS 493, GLY 365, SER 534, ASP 533, ALA 499, GLY 531, THR 501, and LYS 532	
		O sp^3 from CO$_2$H (OH)-N sp^3 from LYS 374	3.042

Ligand	Score/ RMSD (Å)	Group interaction/hydrogen bond	Bond length (Å)
PQ12	−52.44/ 0.06	GLU 418, GLN 421, LYS 374, THR 498, PHE 361, GLY 363, HIS 367, ARG 364, ARG 362, LYS 493, GLY 365, SER 534, ASP 533, ALA 499, GLY 531, THR 501, and LYS 532	
		O sp^3 from CO$_2$H(OH)-N sp^3 from LYS 374	3.155
6ClPQ12	−50.48/ 0.29	GLU 418, GLN 421, GLU 356, LYS 374, THR 498, PHE 361, GLY 363, HIS 367, ARG 364, ARG 362, LYS 493, GLY 365, SER 534, ASP 533, ALA 499, GLY 531, THR 501, and LYS 532	
		O sp^3 from CO$_2$H(OH)-N sp^3 from LYS 374	3.059
		O sp^3 from CO$_2$H(CO)-N sp^3 from LYS 374	3.068
HPQ12	−51.36/ 0.37	GLU 418, GLN 421, LYS 425, SER 423, LYS 374, THR 498, PHE 361, GLY 363, HIS 367, ARG 364, LYS 493, GLY 365, ILE 420, SER 534, ASP 533, ALA 499, GLY 531, THR 501, and LYS 532	
		O sp^3 from CO$_2$H(OH)-N sp^3 from LYS 374	3.112
6MePQ12	−52.57/ 0.03	GLU 418, GLN 421, LYS 374, THR 498, PHE 361, ARG 362, GLY 363, HIS 367, ARG 364, LYS 493, GLY 365, SER 534, ASP 533, ALA 499, GLY 531, THR 501, and LYS 532	
		O sp^3 from CO$_2$H(OH)-N sp^3 from LYS 374	3.046
PQ13	−57.18/ 0.06	LYS 425, GLU 418, GLN 421, LYS 374, THR 498, PHE 361, ARG 362, GLY 363, HIS 367, ARG 364, LYS 493, LEU 360, GLY 365, SER 534, ASP 533, ALA 499, GLY 531, THR 501, and LYS 532	
		O sp^3 from CO$_2$H(OH)-N sp^3 from LYS 374	3.032
6ClPQ13	−58.51/ 0.09	GLU 418, GLN 421, LYS 374, THR 498, PHE 361, ARG 362, GLY 363, HIS 367, ARG 364, LYS 493, GLY 365, SER 534, ASP 533, ALA 499, GLY 531, THR 501, and LYS 532	
		O sp^3 from CO$_2$H(OH)-N sp^3 from LYS 374	3.099
HPQ13	−58.40/ 0.05	ARG 364, LYS 425, GLY 363, ARG 362, TYR 268, GLN 421, GLU 418, PHE 361, ILE 420, ASN 419, LYS 374, ARG 375, ILE 377, LEU 360, MET 263, SER 423, and TRP 416	2.989
		O sp^2 from CO$_2$H(CO)-N sp^3 from LYS 425	
		O sp^3 from CO$_2$H (CO-O sp^3 from SER 423	3.059
		O sp^2 from NO$_2$-N sp^2 from ASN 419	2.969
6MePQ13	−61.22/ 0.04	LYS 425, ARG 364, GLY 365, ASP 533, SER 531, THR 501, ARG 362, PHE 361, LYS 374, LYS 532, GLY 531, ALA 499, HIS 367, THR 498, LYS 493, SER 423, GLN 421, and GLU 418	
		O sp^3 from CO$_2$H(OH)-O sp^2 from GLU 418	2.978
APQ13	−60.00/ 0.06	GLU 418, LYS 425, GLN 421, LYS 374, THR 498, PHE 361, ARG 362, GLY 363, HIS 367, ARG 364, GLY 365, SER 534, ASP 533, ALA 499, GLY 531, THR 501, and LYS 532	
		O sp^3 from CO$_2$H(OH)-N sp^3 from LYS 374	3.008
6ClAPQ13	−57.07/ 0.64	LYS 425, ARG 364, GLU 356, GLY 365, ASP 533, GLY 531, THR 501, ARG 362, GLY 363, PHE 361, LYS 374, LYS 532, ALA 499, HIS 367, LYS 493, SER 534, GLN 421, and GLU 41	
		O sp^3 from CO$_2$H(OH)-N sp^3 from LYS 374	2.934
HAPQ13	−58.14/ 0.07	SER 423, LYS 425, GLN 421, GLU 418, ILE 420, ASN 419, LYS 374, ARG 364, GLY 363, ARG 362, PHE 361, ILE 377, ARG 375, LEU 360, and MET 263	
		O sp^2 from CO$_2$H(CO)-O sp^3 from LYS 425	2.874

Ligand	Score/ RMSD (Å)	Group interaction/hydrogen bond	Bond length (Å)
		O sp^3 from CO$_2$H(CO)-O sp^3 from SER 423	2.994
6MeAPQ13	−56.87/ 0.13	LYS 425, ARG 364, GLY 365, ASP 533, GLY 531, THR 501, ARG 362, GLY 363, THR 498, PHE 361, LYS 374, LYS 532, ALA 499, HIS 367, LYS 493, SER 534, GLN 421, and GLU 418	
		O sp^2 from CO$_2$H(CO)-N sp^3 from LYS 374	3.097

Table 3.
List of docking interactions between the ligand molecules and human DNA topoisomerase I using CLC Drug Discovery Workbench Software.

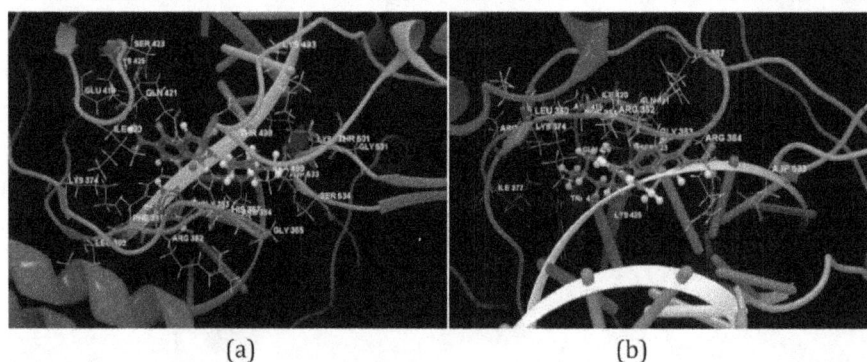

(a) (b)

Figure 9.
(a) Docking pose of 6ClPQ 11 ligand interacting with amino acid residues of the ligand binding site of human DNA topoisomerase I. (b) Docking pose of HPQ11 ligand interacting with amino acid residues of the ligand binding site of human DNA topoisomerase I.

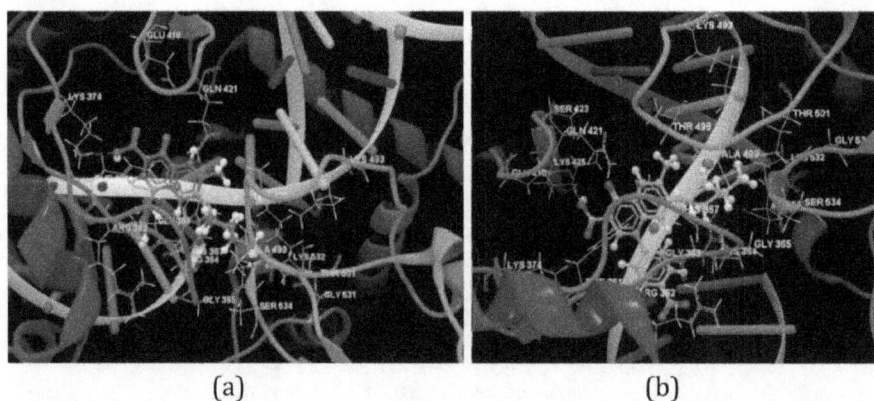

(a) (b)

Figure 10.
(a) Docking pose of 6MePQ11 ligand interacting with amino acid residues of the ligand binding site of human DNA topoisomerase I. (b) Docking pose of 6MePQ13 ligand interacting with amino acid residues of the ligand binding site of human DNA topoisomerase I.

HPQ11, was predicted to have a significant docking score (−49.57) and forms one hydrogen bond with ASP95 (bond length − 3.081 Å) (**Figure 14a**). Docking poses of all quinolone derivatives in the ligand binding site of topoisomerase IV from *Klebsiella pneumoniae* are shown in **Figure 15b**.

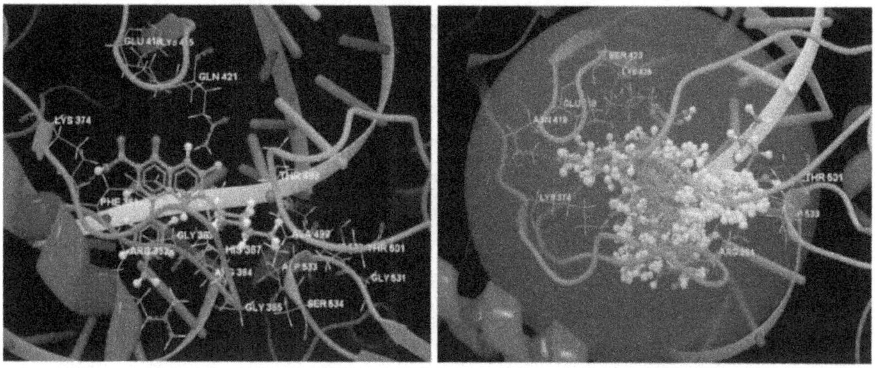

(a) (b)

Figure 11.
(a) Docking pose of APQ13 ligand interacting with amino acid residues of the ligand binding site of human DNA topoisomerase I. (b) Overlay of docking poses of all ligands interacting with amino acid residues of the ligand binding site of human DNA topoisomerase I.

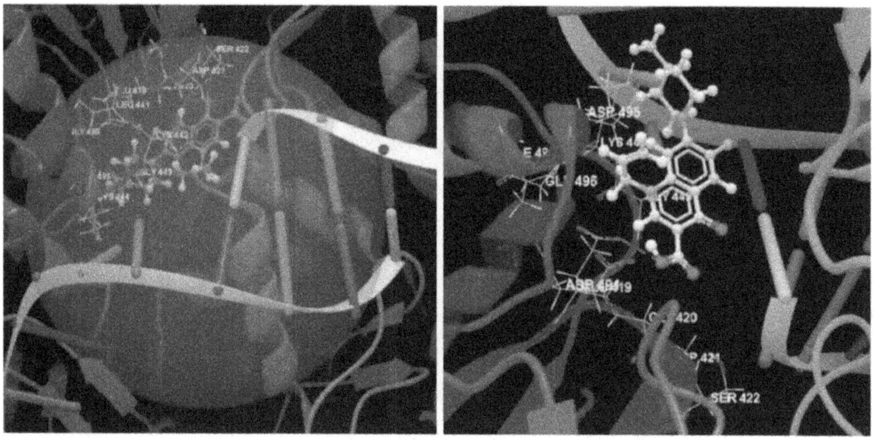

(a) (b)

Figure 12.
(a) Binding site and docking pose of the co-crystallized LFX ligand interacting with the amino acid residues of ligand binding site of the topoisomerase IV. (b) Docking pose of the PQ4 ligand interacting with the amino acid residues of ligand binding site of the topoisomerase IV.

Important molecular properties of the investigated compounds, e.g., molecular weight, flexible bonds, the number of hydrogen bond donors, the number of hydrogen bond acceptors, and log P, have been calculated. These parameters can be used to evaluate whether a molecule has properties that would make it a likely orally active drug, according to the Lipinski's rule of five [22]. The number of violations of the Lipinski rules allows to evaluate drug likeness for a molecule (**Table 5**).

3. Results and discussions

All of the investigated compounds have been docked on human DNA topoisomerase (PDB ID: 1K4T) and topoisomerase IV (PDB ID: 5EIX) from *Klebsiella*

Ligand	Score/ RMSD (Å)	Group interaction/hydrogen bond	Bond length (Å)
LFX	−37.26/0.02	SER 422, ALA 423, ASP 421, GLY 420, LYS 442, LEU 441, GLY 443, GLU 419, LYS 444, ILE 499, GLY 496, and ASP 495	
		O sp^2 from CO-O sp^3 from SER 422	2.590
		O sp^2 from CO-N sp^2 from SER 422	2.856
		O sp^2 from CO-N sp^2 from ASP 421	3.098
		O sp^3 from LVF-N sp^2 from GLY 443	3.344
PQ4	−43.98/0.05	SER 422, ASP 421, GLY 420, GLY 443, GLU 419, ASP 491, LYS 444, ILE 499, GLY 496, and ASP 495	
		O sp^2 from $CO_2H(OH)$-O sp^3 from GLU 419	2.702
6ClPQ4	−41.12/0.25	SER 422, ALA 423, ASP 421, GLY 420, LYS 499, LEU 441, GLY 443, GLU 419, ASP 491, ASP 493, LYS 444, ILE 499, GLY 496, and ASP 495	
		O sp^2 from CO-O sp^3 from SER 422	2.870
		O sp^2 from CO-N sp^2 from SER 422	3.162
HPQ4	−40.60/0.20	SER 422, ASP 421, GLY 420, GLY 443, GLU 419, ASP 491, LYS 444, ILE 499, GLY 496, and ASP 495	
		O sp^2 from $CO_2H(OH)$-O sp^3 from GLU 419	2.880
6MePQ4	−35.70/0.36	SER 422, ASP 421, GLY 420, GLY 443, GLU 419, ASP 491, LYS 444, ILE 499, GLY 496, and ASP 495	
		O sp^2 from $CO_2H(OH)$-O sp^3 from GLU 419	2.911
PQ11	−48.32/0.10	LYS 444, ILE 499, ASP 495, ASP 493, GLY 443, LEU 441, GLU 419, ASP 491, GLY 420, LYS 442, ASP 421, LEU 567, ALA, 423, SER 422, and GLY 568	
		O sp^2 from $CO_2H(OH)$-O sp^2 from ASP 491	2.974
		O sp^2 from CO_2H (OH)-O sp^2 from GLU 419	2.606
		O sp^2 from CO-O sp^3 from SER 422	2.650
6ClPQ11	−41.14/0.28	SER 422, ASP 421, GLY 420, LYS 442, LEU 441, GLY 443, GLU 419, LYS 444, ILE 499, GLY 496, and ASP 495	
		O sp^2 from $CO_2H(CO)$-N sp^2 from ASP 421	3.062
HPQ11	−49.57/0.11	HIS 1077, ASP 421, GLY 420, ASP 493, LYS 442, LEU 441, GLU 419, GLY 443, LYS 444, ILE 499, ILE 445, ASP 495, and ARG 1029	
		O sp^2 from $CO_2H(OH)$-N sp^2 from ASP 495	3.081
6MePQ11	−39.64/0.18	SER 422, HIS 1077 ASP 421, GLY 420, ASP 491, ASP 493, LYS 442, LEU 441, GLU 419, GLY 443, LYS 444, ILE 499, ASP 495, ARG 1029, and ILE 445	
		O sp^2 from CO_2H (OH)-N sp^2 from ASP 495	3.088
PQ12	−42.76/0.18	HIS 1077, GLY 420, ASP 493, LYS 442, LEU 441, GLU 419, GLY 443, LYS 444, ILE 499, ILE 445, ASP 495, ASP 491, ARG 1029, and GLY 496	
		O sp^2 from $CO_2H(OH)$-O sp^2 from ASP 493	2.571
		O sp^2 from CO_2H (OH)-O sp^2 from GLU 419	3.135
6ClPQ12	−35.34/0.07	SER 422, ALA 423, ASP 491, ASP 421, GLY 420, LYS 442, LEU 441, GLY 443, GLU 419, LYS 444, ILE 499, GLY 496, and ASP 495	
		O sp^2 from CO-O sp^3 from SER 422	2.942
		O sp^2 from CO-N sp^2 from SER 422	3.185
HPQ12	−40.45/0.13	SER 422, ALA 423, ASP 421, GLY 420, LYS 442, LEU 441, GLY 443, GLU 419, LYS 444, ILE 499, GLY 496, and ASP 495	
		O sp^2 from CO-O sp^3 from SER 422	2.993
		O sp^2 from CO-N sp^2 from SER 422	3.060
		O sp^2 from CO-N sp^2 from ASP 421	3.159

Ligand	Score/ RMSD (Å)	Group interaction/hydrogen bond	Bond length (Å)
6MePQ12	−35.39/0.17	SER 422, ALA 423, ASP 421, ASP 491, GLY 420, LYS 442, LEU 441, GLY 443, GLU 419, LYS 444, ILE 499, GLY 496, and ASP 495	
		O sp^2 from CO-O sp^3 from SER 422	2.943
		O sp^2 from CO-N sp^2 from SER 422	3.156
PQ13	−38.74/0.19	SER 422, ASP 421, ASP 4921, GLY 420, LYS 422, LEU 441, GLY 443, GLU 419, LYS 444, ILE 499, ASP 495, ARG 1029, HIS 1077, SER 1080, ASP 1079, GLY 1079, and HIS 1075	
		O sp^2 from CO-N sp^2 from ARG 1029	2.963
		O sp^2 from CO_2H (OH)-N sp^2 from ARG 1029	3.081
		O sp^2 from NO_2-O sp^2 from SER 1080	2.489
6ClPQ13	−37.47/0.32	SER 422, ALA 423, ASP 421, GLY 420, ASP 493, ASP 491, LEU 441, GLY 443, GLU 419, LYS 444, ILE 499, GLY 496, and ASP 495	
		O sp^3 from CO-O sp^3 from SER 422	2.664
		O sp^2 from CO-N sp^2 from SER 422	2.817
		O sp^2 from CO-N sp^2 from ASP 421	3.253
HPQ13	−40.08/0.05	HIS 1075, ASP 1079, CYS 1082, VAL 1041, GLY 1078, HIS 1077, SER 1080, ALA 1081, ARG 1029, LYS 444, ILE 499, ASP 495, ASP 493, GLU 419, LEU, 441, GLY 496, LYS 442, and GLY 443	
		O sp^2 from CO_2H(OH)-N sp^2 from CYS 1082	3.241
		O sp^2 from CO_2H (OH)-O sp^2 from GLY 1078	2.876
6MePQ13	−37.58/0.45	SER 422, ALA 423, ASP 421, ASP 493, ASP 491, GLY 420, LYS 442, LEU 441, GLY 443, GLU 419, LYS 444, ILE 499, and ASP 495	
		O sp^2 from CO-O sp^3 from SER 422	2.797
		O sp^2 from CO-N sp^2 from SER 422	2.926
		O sp^2 from CO-N sp^2 from ASP 421	3.247
APQ13	−42.96/0.32	SER 422, ASP 421, ASP 493, GLY 420, LYS 442, LEU 441, GLY 443, GLU 419, ILE 499, ASP 495, ILE 445, ARG 1029, and HIS 1077	
		O sp^2 from CO_2H(OH)-N sp^2 from ARG 1029	2.820
		O sp^2 from CO_2H(OH)-O sp^2 from ASP 495	3.113
		O sp^2 from CO_2H (OH)-O sp^2 from ASP 495	3.052
		N sp^3 from NH_2-O sp^2 from GLU 419	2.922
		N sp^3 from NH_2-N sp^2 from GLY 443	3.052
6ClAPQ13	−39.93/0.40	ASP 421, GLY 420, LYS 442, LEU 441, GLY 443, GLU 419, ILE 499, ILE 445, LYS 444, ASP 495, ARG 1029, and HIS 1077	
		O sp^2 from COOH(CO)-N sp^2 from ARG 1029	3.063
		O sp^2 from COOH(OH)-O sp^2 from ASP 495	3.132
		N sp^3 from NH_2-O sp^2 from GLU 419	2.706
		N sp^3 from NH_2-N sp^2 from GLY 443	3.137
HAPQ13	−37.50/0.50	HIS 1077, ARG 1029, LYS 444, ILE 445, ILE 499, ASP 495, ASP 421, GLU 419, LEU, 441, GLY 420, LYS 442, and GLY 443	
		O sp^2 from CO_2H(OH)-N sp^2 from ARG 1029	2.851
		O sp^2 from CO_2H(OH)-O sp^2 from ASP 495	3.199
		N sp^3 from NH_2-O sp^2 from GLU 419	2.707
		N sp^3 from NH_2-N sp^2 from GLY 443	3.150

Ligand	Score/ RMSD (Å)	Group interaction/hydrogen bond	Bond length (Å)
6MeAPQ13	−39.85/0.20	ASP 421, GLY 420, LYS 442, LEU 441, GLU 419, GLY 443, ILE 499, ILE 445, LYS 444, ASP 495, ARG 1029, and HIS 1077	
		O sp^2 from CO$_2$H(CO)-N sp^2 from ARG 1029	3.154
		O sp^2 from CO$_2$H(OH)-O sp^2 from ASP 495	3.115
		O sp^2 from CO$_2$H(OH)-O sp^2 from ASP 495	3.252
		N sp^3 from NH$_2$-O sp^2 from GLU 419	2.705
		N sp^3 from NH$_2$-N sp^2 from GLY 443	3.132

Table 4.
List of docking interactions between the ligand molecules and topoisomerase IV (PDB ID: 5EIX) from Klebsiella pneumoniae *using CLC Drug Discovery Workbench Software.*

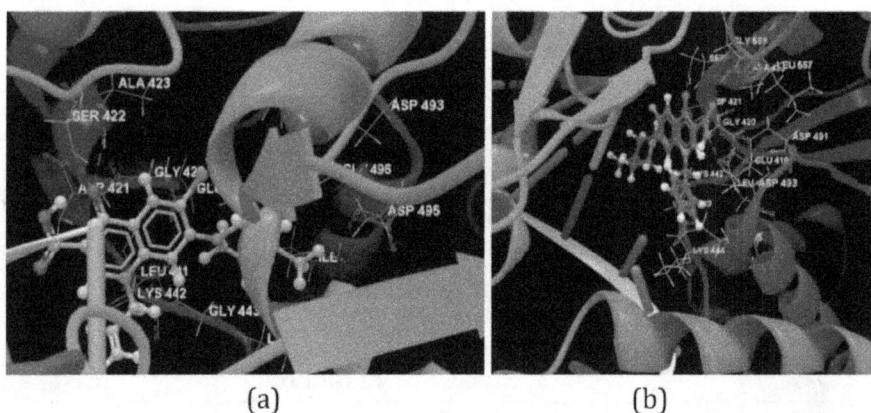

(a)　　　　　　　　　　(b)

Figure 13.
(a) Docking pose of 6ClPQ4 ligand interacting with amino acid residues of ligand binding site of the topoisomerase IV. (b) Docking pose of PQ11 ligand interacting with amino acid residues of ligand binding site of the topoisomerase IV.

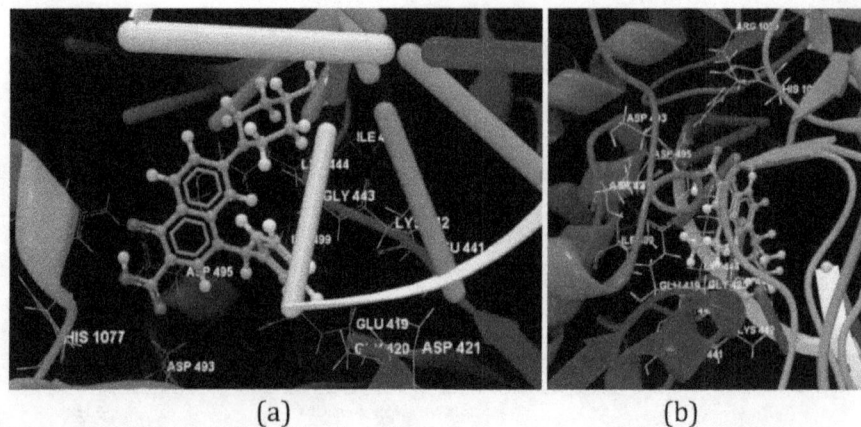

(a)　　　　　　　　　　(b)

Figure 14.
(a) Docking pose of HPQ11 ligand interacting with amino acid residues of ligand binding site of the topoisomerase IV. (b) Docking pose of PQ12 ligand interacting with amino acid residues of ligand binding site of the topoisomerase IV.

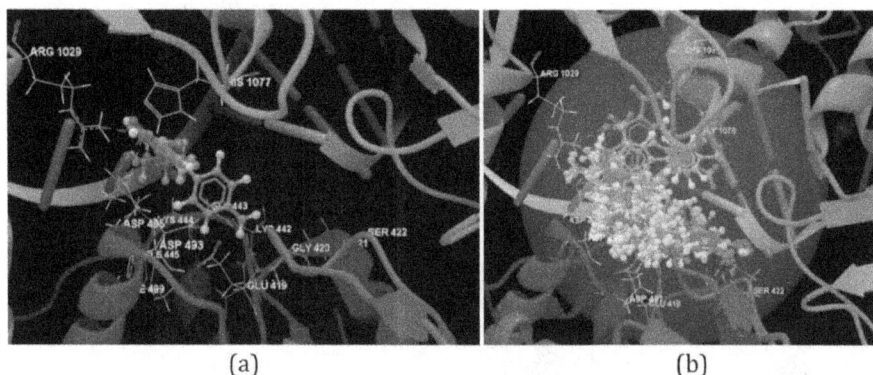

(a)

(b)

Figure 15.
(a) Docking pose of APQ13 ligand interacting with amino acid residues of ligand binding site of the topoisomerase IV. (b) Overlay of docking poses of all ligands interacting with amino acid residues of ligand binding site of the topoisomerase IV.

Ligands	Atoms	Weight (Daltons)	Flexible bonds	Lipinski violations (a) (b)	Hydrogen donors	Hydrogen acceptors	Log P (a) (b)
TTC	51	418.42	3	0 —	2	8	3.55 —
LFX	45	360.36	2	— 0	1	7	— 1.26
PQ4	46	344.38	4	1 1	1	5	5.34 5.67
6ClPQ4	46	360.83	4	1 1	1	5	5.87 6.20
HPQ4	46	326.39	4	1 1	1	5	5.24 5.57
6MePQ4	49	340.42	4	1 1	1	5	5.60 5.94
PQ11	52	394.44	4	1 1	1	5	5.99 6.52
6ClPQ11	52	410.89	4	1 1	1	5	6.52 7.05
HPQ11	52	376.45	4	1 1	1	5	5.89 6.42
6MePQ11	55	390.47	4	1 1	1	5	6.25 6.78
PQ12	48	346.40	3	1 1	1	5	5.10 5.63
6ClPQ12	48	362.85	3	1 1	1	5	5.63 6.16
HPQ12	48	328.41	3	0 1	1	5	5.00 5.53
6MePQ12	51	342.43	3	1 1	1	5	5.36 5.89
PQ13	51	425.41	4	1 1	1	8	6.08 6.42
6ClPQ13	51	441.86	4	1 1	1	8	6.61 6.94
HPQ13	51	407.42	4	1 1	1	8	5.98 6.31
6MePQ13	54	421.45	4	1 1	1	8	6.35 6.68
APQ13	51	395.43	3	1 1	3	6	5.37 5.90
6ClAPQ13	51	411.88	3	1 1	3	6	5.90 6.43
HAPQ13	51	377.44	3	1 1	3	6	5.27 5.80
6MeAPQ13	54	391.46	3	1 1	3	6	5.63 6.17

(a) For protein receptor PDB ID: 1K4T.
(b) For protein receptor PDB ID: 5EIX.

Table 5.
Ligands with various properties.

Score

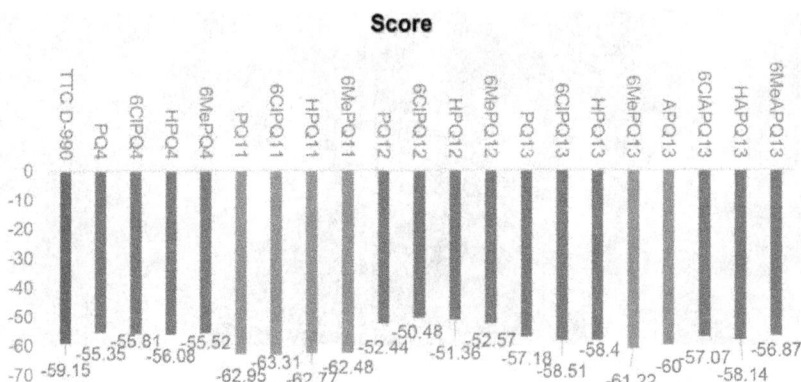

Figure 16.
Docking scores of the investigated quinolone compounds targeting human DNA topoisomerase I (PDB ID: 1K4T).

Score

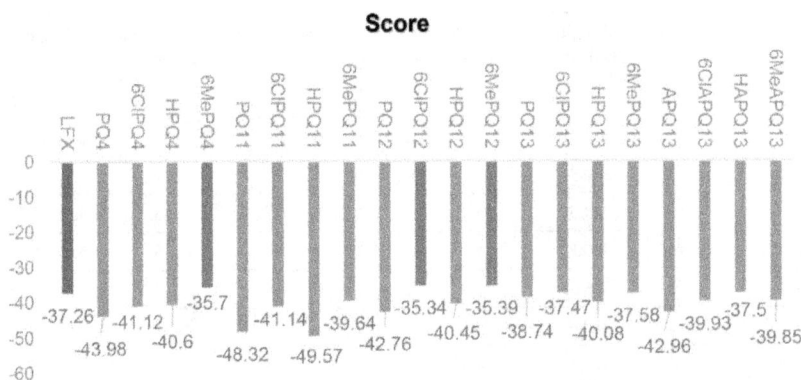

Figure 17.
Docking scores of the investigated quinolone compounds targeting topoisomerase IV (PDB ID: 5EIX) from Klebsiella pneumoniae.

pneumoniae. In case of the molecular docking studies on the human DNA topoisomerase I, all the quinolone derivatives reveal docking scores greater than -50. Only five compounds, e.g., PQ11 (-63.31), 6ClPQ11 (-62.95), HPQ11 (-62.77), 6MePQ11 (-62.48), and 6MePQ13 (-61.22), reveal better docking scores than that of co-crystallized TTC (-59.15) (**Figure 16**). In case of the molecular docking studies on topoisomerase IV from *Klebsiella pneumoniae*, only three quinolone derivatives, e.g., 6MePQ4 (-35.7), 6ClPQ12 (-35.34), and 6MePQ12 (-35.39), reveal docking scores less than that of levofloxacin (-37.26). The compounds that show better docking scores than that of levofloxacin are HPQ11 (-49.57), PQ11 (-48.32), PQ4 (-43.98), PQ12 (-42.76), APQ13 (-42.96), and 6ClPQ4 (-41.12) (**Figure 17**). It was observed that the presence of the benzyl substituent in N-1 position of the 7(4-methyl-piperidinyl)-quinolones core leads to increased docking score against human DNA topoisomerase and topoisomerase IV from *Klebsiella pneumoniae*. The compounds PQ11, 6ClPQ11, HPQ11, and 6MePQ11 reveal better docking scores than that of the reference ligands, topotecan (TTC) and levofloxacin (LFX), docked on human DNA topoisomerase (PDB ID:1K4T) and topoisomerase IV (PDB ID: 5EIX) from *Klebsiella pneumoniae*, respectively.

4. Conclusions

The virtual screening of the investigated compounds using docking has been carried out with CLC Drug Discovery Workbench Software and has led to the identification of quinolone derivatives for inhibiting the activities of topoisomerase I and topoisomerase IV. It was observed that the presence of the benzyl substituent in N1 position of the 7-(4-methyl-piperidinyl)-quinolones core leads to increased docking score against human DNA topoisomerase and topoisomerase IV from *Klebsiella pneumoniae.*

The compounds PQ11 (1-benzyl-6-fluoro-7-(4-methyl-piperidin-1-yl)-1,4-dihydro-4-oxo-quinolin-3-carboxylic acid), 6ClPQ11 (1-benzyl-6-chloro-7-(4-methyl-piperidin-1-yl)-1,4-dihydro-4-oxo-quinolin-3-carboxylic acid), HPQ11 (1-benzyl-7-(4-methyl-piperidin-1-yl)-1,4-dihydro-4-oxo-quinolin-3-carboxylic acid), and 6MePQ11 (1-benzyl-6-methyl-7-(4-methyl-piperidin-1-yl)-1,4-dihydro-4-oxo-quinolin-3-carboxylic acid) reveal better docking scores than that of the reference ligands, topotecan (TTC) and levofloxacin (LFX), docked on human DNA topoisomerase (PDB ID: 1K4T) and topoisomerase IV (PDB ID: 5EIX) from *Klebsiella pneumoniae,* respectively.

Acknowledgements

This chapter has been financed through the NUCLEU Program, which is implemented with the support of Ministry of Research and Innovation (MCI), project no. 19-41 01 02.

Conflict of interest

The authors declare no conflict of interest.

Author details

Lucia Pintilie* and Amalia Stefaniu
National Institute of Chemical-Pharmaceutical Research and Development, Bucharest, Romania

*Address all correspondence to: lucia.pintilie@gmail.com

IntechOpen

References

[1] Pintilie L. Quinolones: Synthesis and antibacterial activity. In: Bobbarala V, editor. Antimicrobial Agents. Rijeka: Intech; 2012. pp. 255-272. DOI: 10.5772/33215

[2] Pintilie L. Quinolone compounds with activity against multidrug-resistant gram-positive microorganisms. In: Bobbarala V, editor. Concepts, Compounds and the Alternatives of Antibacterials. Rijeka: Intech; 2015. pp. 45-80. DOI: 10.5772/60948

[3] Advani RH, Hurwitz HI, Gordon MS, Ebbinghaus SW, Mendelson DS, Wakelee HA, et al. Voreloxin, a first-in-class anticancer quinolone derivative, in relapsed/refractory solid tumors: A report on two dosing schedules. Clinical Cancer Research. 2010;16:2167-2175. DOI: 10.1158/1078-0432.CCR-09-2236

[4] Hawtin RE, Stockett DE, Byl JAW, McDowell RS, Tan N, Michelle R, et al. Voreloxin is an anticancer quinolone derivative that intercalates DNA and poisons topoisomerase II. PLoS One. 2010;5:e10186. DOI: 10.1371/journal.pone.0010186

[5] Jiar X-D, Wang S, Wang M-H, Xia G-M, Liu X-J, Chai Y, et al. Synthesis and *in vitro* antitumor activity of novel naphthyridinone derivatives. Chinese Chemical Letters. 2017;28:235-239. DOI: 10.1016/j.cclet.2016.07.024

[6] Khalil OM, Gedawy EM, El-Malah AA, Adly ME. Novel nalidixic acid derivatives targeting topoisomerase II enzyme; design, synthesis, anticancer activity and effect on cell cycle profile. Bioorganic Chemistry. 2019;83:262-276. DOI: 10.1016/j.bioorg.2018.10.058

[7] Dong Y, Xu C, Zhao X, Domagala J, Drlica K. Fluoroquinolone action against mycobacteria: Effects of C-8 substituents on growth, survival, and resistance. Antimicrobial Agents and Chemotherapy. 1998;42:2978-2984. DOI: 10.1128/AAC.42.11.2978

[8] Aubry A, Pan XS, Fisher LM, Jarlier V, Cambau E. Mycobacterium tuberculosis DNA Gyrase: Interaction with quinolones and correlation with Antimycobacterial drug activity. Antimicrobial Agents and Chemotherapy. 2004;48:1281-1288. DOI: 10.1128/AAC.48.4.1281-1288.2004

[9] Kishii R, Yamaguchi Y, Takei M. *In Vitro* activities and Spectrum of the novel Fluoroquinolone Lascufloxacin (KRP-AM1977). Antimicrobial Agents and Chemotherapy. 2017;61:e-00120-17. DOI: 10.1128/AAC.00120-17

[10] Murata M, Kosai K, Yamauchi S, Sasaki D, Kaku N, Uno N, et al. *In Vitro* activity of Lascufloxacin against *Streptococcus pneumoniae* with mutations in the quinolone resistance-determining regions. Antimicrobial Agents and Chemotherapy. 2018;62:30197-30117. DOI: 10.1128/AAC.01971-17

[11] Walsh CT, Wencewicz TA. Prospects for new antibiotics: A molecule-centered perspective. The Journal of Antibiotics. 2014;67:7-22 https://doi.org/10.1038/ja.2013.49

[12] Flick AC, Ding HX, Leverett CA, Fink SJ, O'Donnell CJ. Synthetic approaches to new drugs approved during 2016. Journal of Medicinal Chemistry. 2018;61:7004-7031. DOI: 10.1021/acs.jmedchem.8b00260

[13] CLC Drug Discovery Workbench. Available from: http://www.clcbio.com

[14] Pintilie L, Oniscu C, Voiculescu G, Draghici C, Caproiu MT, Alexandru N, et al. Synthesis and antibacterial activity of some novel fluoroquinolones. Romanian Biotechnological Letters. 2003;8:1197-1204

[15] Pintilie L, Oniscu C, Voiculescu G, Draghici C, Caproiu MT, Alexandru N, et al. Synthesis of some novel desfluoroquinolones. Romanian Biotechnological Letters. 2003;**8**: 1303-1309

[16] Pintilie L, Oniscu C, Draghici C, Caproiu MT, Alexandru N, Damian E, et al. 6 methyl-quinolones with biological activity. Romanian Biotechnological Letters. 2003;**8**: 1163-1168

[17] Pintilie L, Negut C, Oniscu C, Caproiu MT, Nechifor M. Synthesis and antibacterial activity of some novel desfluoroquinolones. Revista de Chimie. 2009;**60**:871-975

[18] Pintilie L, Negut C, Oniscu C, Caproiu MT, Nechifor M, Iancu L, et al. Synthesis and antibacterial activity of some novel quinolones. Romanian Biotechnological Letters. 2009;**14**: 4756-4767

[19] Pintilie L, Tanase C. RO Patent application RO A/00767; 02.10.2018

[20] Pintilie L, Nita S. RO 128027-B1/ 28.02.2018

[21] Spartan'14 Wavefunction, Inc. Irvine, CA. Available from www. wavefun.com

[22] Pintilie L, Stefaniu A. Docking studies on novel analogues of 8-chloro-quinolones against *Staphylococcus aureus*. In: Vlachakis DP, editor. Molecular Docking. Rijeka: Intech; 2018. pp. 77-98. DOI: 10.5772/ intechopen.72995

[23] Staker BL, Hjerrild K, Feese MD, Behnke CA, Burgin AB Jr, Stewart L. The mechanism of topoisomerase I poisoning by a camptothecin analog. PNAS. 2002;**26**: 15387-15392. DOI: 10.1073/ pnas.242259599

[24] Veselkov DA, Laponogov I, Pan X-S, Selvarajah J, Skamrova GB, Branstrom A, et al. Structure of a quinolone-stabilized cleavage complex of topoisomerase IV from *Klebsiella pneumoniae* and comparison with a related *Streptococcus pneumoniae* complex. Acta Cryst. 2016;**D72**:488-496. DOI: 10.1107/S2059798316001212

Virtual Screening of Sesquiterpenoid *Pogostemon herba* as Predicted Cyclooxygenase Inhibitor

Sentot Joko Raharjo

Abstract

To analyze the structural features that dictate the selectivity of the two isoforms of the cyclooxygenase (COX), the three-dimensional structure of COX-1/COX-2 was assessed by means of binding energy calculation by way of virtual molecular dynamic simulations using ligand sesquiterpenoid Pogostemon herba. This study was conducted to investigate the molecular interaction between ligand alpha-bulnesene (CID94275), alpha-guaiene (CID197152), seychellene (CID519743), and alpha-patchouli alcohol isomers (CID442384, CID521903, CID6432585, CID3080622, CID10955174, and CID56928117) to COX-1 and COX-2. Molecular docking tools proposed by Hex 8.0 were employed in this research. Discovery Studio Client 3.5 software tool and virtual molecular dynamic 1.9.1 software were also used to visualize the molecular interactions identified in this research. In order to calculate the binding energy of the molecular dynamic interaction, AMBER12 software was utilized. Results of the analysis on all sesquiterpenoid indicate that those compounds were the inhibitors of COX-1 and COX-2. Overall, the binding energy calculations (using PBSA Model Solvent) of alpha-patchouli alcohol (CID521903) and seychellene (CID519743) have been identified as the candidates of non-selective inhibitor; alpha-bulnesene (CID94275), alpha-guaiene (CID107152), and alpha-patchouli alcohol isomers (CID6432585, CID3080622, CID10955174, CID56928117) have been suggested as the candidates for a selective COX-1 inhibitor; whereas alpha-patchouli alcohol (CID442384) was the candidate for a selective COX-2 inhibitor.

Keywords: molecular dynamic, molecular docking, screening, sesquiterpenoid, sesquiterpenoid alcohol, *pogostemon herba*, alpha-bulnesene, alpha-guaiene, seychellene, alpha-patchouli alcohol isomers, cyclooxygenase, protein COX-1/COX-2, binding energy, scoring

1. Introduction

The rapid development of high-performance computing intensifies the competition to invent faster supercomputers which invention is considered as a national pride. High-performance computing machines are highly valued for having adequate ability to solve complex problems related to national interests in several sectors including national defense, energy, financial sectors and science. Within the global economic growth competition and the advancement in science and technology including the advancement in biology, chemistry, pharmacy and medicine, supercomputers play key roles. In-silico analysis has been developed as the computational approach [1, 2].

Molecular interactions including protein-nucleic acid, drug-protein, protein-protein, enzyme-substrate, and drug-nucleic acid play important roles in many essential biological processes, such as enzyme inhibition, signal transduction, antibody-antigen recognition, transport, gene expression control, cell regulation, up to multi-domain proteins assembly. Stable protein-protein or protein-ligand complexes are often produced by the interaction which complexes are considered essential in performing their biological functions. To determine the binding mode and affinity between interacting molecules, tertiary structure of proteins should be first identified. Unfortunately, conducting experiments to obtain complex structures has been considered challenging and expensive because the experiments would require X-ray crystallography or NMR. Docking computation has been considered a feasible and important approach to comprehend the protein–protein or protein-ligand interactions [3]. Experimental technique has been frequently used to determine the three-dimensional protein structures—and structure of the databases such as Protein Data Bank (PDB) and Worldwide Protein Data Bank. A total of 88,000 protein structures have been identified and most of them are significant in critical metabolic pathways which might be regarded as potential therapeutic target. Therefore, specific databases that contain binary complexes structures would be available, along with information about binding affinities, such as in PDBBIND, PLD, AffinDB and BindDB, molecular docking procedures improvement [3, 4].

In silico virtual screening is a popular identification technique used in in drug discovery projects which distinguishes true actives from inactive or decoy molecules effectively. To have better comprehension on the dynamic behavior of protein drug targets, compound databases can be screened against an ensemble of protein conformations through experiments or generated-computation [5]. Screening states include ligand preparation, protein targets, molecular docking, visualization, binding energy calculation, and scoring [6]. A computer simulation procedure in the form of molecular docking is commonly used to predict the conformation of certain receptor-ligand complex, which receptor is usually a protein or a nucleic acid molecule or the ligands in the form of a small molecule or other protein, or sesquiterpenoid/sesquiterpenoid alcohol interaction to protein cyclooxygenase, as shown **Figure 1**. In modern structure-based drug design, accurate prediction is necessary to determine the binding modes between the ligand and protein. Virtual screening is the most popular docking application that selects molecules from an existing database for further research. As the demand on this computational method keeps increasing, people expected a fast and reliable method. Another application used in this study was molecular complexes investigation [3, 6–11]. Previous studies have shown that dynamic molecular-generated conformations play considerable role in the identification of novel hit compounds because structural

Ligand	Protein	Ligand-Protein Complex	Energy

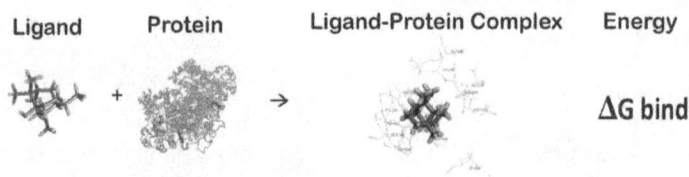

ΔG bind

Figure 1.
Molecular docking-Molecular dynamic ligand to protein.

rearrangements obtained from molecular dynamic show novel-targetable areas. However, predicting the priori is still considered difficult, especially when a molecular dynamic conformation outperforms a virtual screening against the crystal structure.

This study evaluated whether molecular dynamic conformations lead to better virtual screening performance for nine ligand sesquiterpenoid/sesquiterpenoid *Pogostemon herba* to protein cyclooxygenase (COX-1/COX-2). The results of in silico analysis data will be completed with IC_{50} value determination and in-vitro and in-vivo evaluation of the biological activity.

2. Theory of docking and virtual molecular dynamic

Within the process of living system, protein-ligand interactions have been known to play central roles. It has been considered interesting to obtain more comprehensive understanding of protein interactions with small molecules because it leads to better understanding of various functions and therapeutic intervention. As a matter of fact, molecular recognition is a complex interplay of several factors including inter-molecular interactions of protein, ligand and the surrounding solvent, conformational variations of binding partners and the thermodynamics of molecular association. The non-covalent reversible binding of small-molecules to proteins also plays a central role in the field of biology. Several processes are known crucial in living systems that involve specific recognition of small molecule ligands by proteins. For instance, certain enzymes affect their substrates and catalyze chemical reactions inside the cells, where transporters recognize specific molecules based on the movement across membrane barriers, receptors that are specifically bind to hormones or other chemical messengers for inter- and intracellular communication. Finally, antibodies uniquely can bind to other chemical agents to mount vital defense mechanisms against infections and diseases. In general, protein-ligand binding in an aqueous environment is described as follows.

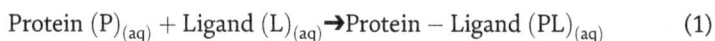

$$\text{Protein (P)}_{(aq)} + \text{Ligand (L)}_{(aq)} \rightarrow \text{Protein} - \text{Ligand (PL)}_{(aq)} \qquad (1)$$

A change in the free energy (ΔG) is always followed by chemical reactions and change in two other important quantities; enthalpy (ΔH)—the heat content and entropy (ΔS) that showed disorder of temperature-independent degree. The relationship between these quantities is shown as follows:

$$\Delta G^{\circ} = \Delta H - T\Delta S \qquad (2)$$

Some factors including electrostatic and van der Waals interactions, ionization effects, conformational changes and the role of solvent affect the changes in the binding of free energy. Those factors are manifested as either favorable or unfavorable changes in entropy and enthalpy. In order to create a spontaneous reaction, the free energy change should be negative at equilibrium, ΔG° which relates to the equilibrium constant (K) in this following expression:

$$\Delta G^{\circ} = -RT\ln K \qquad (3)$$

where R is the gas constant and T is the absolute temperature. Using this relationship, free energy changes can be derived from experimentally measurable quantity, K. Biological K values exhibit a wide range from weak to very strong binding.

Scoring function in ligand-protein docking is expected to identify the preferred binding poses of ligands. However, considering the computational efficiency, approximations were usually introduced into the scoring functions, which unfortunately, often impair the prediction accuracy [12]. The scoring functions of ligand–protein docking can be roughly categorized into two classes: force field-based scoring functions and knowledge-based scoring functions. A force field-based scoring consists of a few potential terms, such as van der Waals interactions, electrostatic interactions, hydrophobic effects, desolvation energies, and entropic effects, and the total energy of a conformation is calculated by summing up the contributions of all energy terms [13, 14].

Inter-atomic interactions mediate the non-covalent binding of small-molecule ligand to proteins. The interactions usually include electrostatic and van der Waals interactions (**Figure 2**). The affinity of receptor-ligand binding is strongly determined by other factors such as entropy, desolvation, flexibility of receptor structure and the structural water molecules in the binding site [15, 16]. A brief literature review of the importance of protein-ligand interactions and other factors contributing to binding affinity is described as follows.

Protein-ligand electrostatic complementarity and the ligand at the binding interface are both vital for the formation of complex. The predominant types of electrostatic interactions appear in the form of hydrogen bonding, salt bridges, and metal interactions.

As the most important directional interaction in biological macromolecules, hydrogen bonding is known for conferring stability to protein structure and selectivity to protein-ligand interactions [17]. Hydrogen bonding normally occurs between two electronegative atoms, which donor is covalently bound to hydrogen atom, while the acceptor contains a lone pair of electrons. The attractive interaction between partial positive charge in the hydrogen atom and partial negative charge on the acceptor atom forms strong electrostatic attraction. Several theoretical and experimental studies have successfully confirmed an additional covalent component to hydrogen bonds based empty σ^* anti- bonding orbital of the hydrogen atom and highest occupied orbital of the acceptor interaction [17, 18]. In hydrophobic interactions, non-polar parts of the molecule interact (**Figure 2**). The non-polar parts of protein-ligand complexes at the interacting surfaces are covered by the binding causing water molecules displacement which eventually increases the

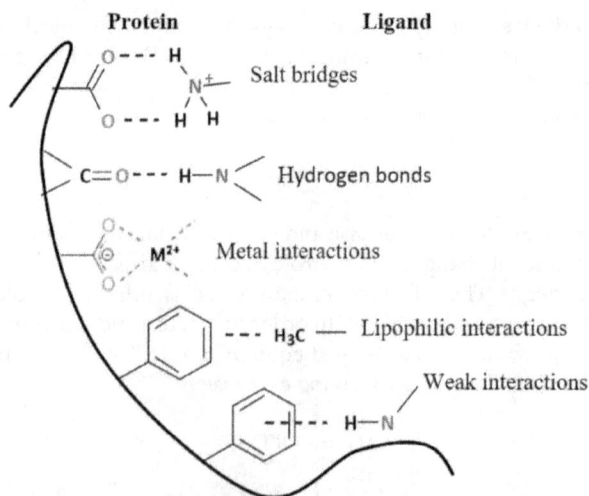

Figure 2.
Major type of non-bonded interactions in protein-ligand complexes [17].

entropy. Hydrophobic interactions are entropy-driven and they play crucial roles in ligand binding [16, 18].

Finding an accurate modeling of protein-ligand binding is an extremely challenging task due to its complexity. Usually, thermodynamics and statistical mechanical principles are employed to develop relatively accurate, but computationally demanding treatment of protein-ligand interactions. In this method, full-scale molecular dynamic simulation using explicit solvent and flexible protein and ligand molecules is employed [15, 17]. Both, absolute and relative binding energy can be measured using free energy approach. The absolute binding free energy method which has been considered an accurate method; it involves separate simulation treatment for solvated protein, ligand and the complex. Prior information is not quite necessary regarding the structure and binding affinity of the complex. A well-known structure for the complex is used within the context of relative free energy calculation as a reference, while the gaps in binding free energy are measured for the ligand of interest. Measurement can be carried out in the form of alchemical transformation of reference ligand into target ligand. Molecular dynamics is used in exhaustive sampling of the configuration space. The accuracy of these methods is determined by the underlying atomic force field and proper selection of protocol to address certain problem at hand [17, 18].

Scoring functions are based on knowledge focus on the optimization of specified terms and they use other optimization methods to set the best weighing for each scoring term regarding the training sets. Hence, these methods are often called as informatics-driven methods including IFACE [19, 20], DARS [21], SPA-PP [22], DrugScorePPI [23], TS [24], etc. In the past decades, free energy perturbation (FEP) [25] as well as energy representation (ER) [21] that are more theoretically rigorous free energy calculation methods, has emerged. Molecular Mechanics/Poisson Boltzmann Surface Area (MM/PBSA) [26] and Molecular mechanics/generalized Born surface area (MM/GBSA) [27] are commonly employed to estimate ligand-protein binding free energies. Unfortunately, these methods are rather time-consuming compared to other scoring functions. Yet, rapid advancement of computer hardware technology seems promising, and it is expected to allow these methods to be used in protein-protein docking in the near future.

The MM/PBSA and MM/GBSA approaches are more computationally efficient when they were compared to thermodynamic integration (TI) and free energy perturbation (FEP) approaches. Besides, they allow decomposition into different interaction terms to occur [13, 26, 28]. MM/PBSA and MM/GBSA are more efficient in tem of computation. Another similar approach is the linear interaction energy (LIE) method, which calculates the average energy interaction in MD simulations to estimate the absolute binding free energy. Similarly, LIE restricts the simulations only to two end points of ligand binding. Different from most molecular docking empirical scoring functions, MM/PBSA and MM/GBSA do not demand a large training set to fit different parameters for each energy term [25]. In addition, MM/PBSA and MM/GBSA allow rigorous free energy decomposition into contributions to occur, originating from different groups of atoms or types of interaction [29, 30]. The binding free energy (ΔG_{bind}) between a ligand and a receptor protein offered in these methods to form a complex Receptor protein - Ligand is calculated as follows.

$$\Delta G_{bind} = G_{complex} \left(G_{protein} + G_{ligand} \right) \quad (4)$$

$$\Delta G_{bind} = \Delta H - T\Delta S \char`~ \Delta E_{MM} + \Delta G_{sol} - T\Delta S \quad (5)$$

$$\Delta E_{MM} = \Delta E_{internal} + \Delta E_{electrostatic} + \Delta E_{vdW} \quad (6)$$

$$\Delta G_{sol} = \Delta G_{PB/GB} + \Delta G_{SA} \quad (7)$$

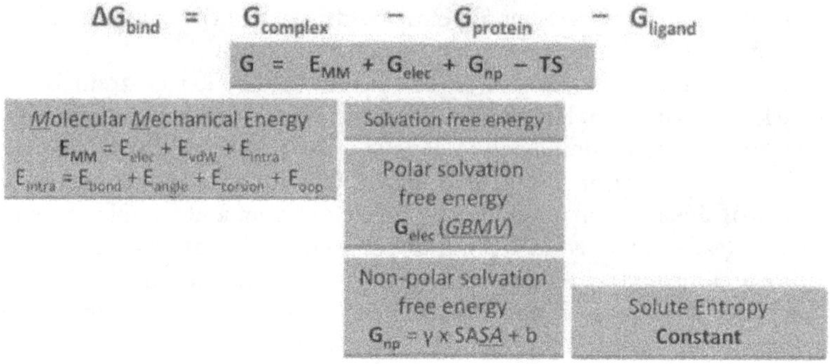

$$\Delta G_{bind} = G_{complex} - G_{protein} - G_{ligand}$$

$$G = E_{MM} + G_{elec} + G_{np} - TS$$

Molecular Mechanical Energy
$E_{MM} = E_{elec} + E_{vdW} + E_{intra}$
$E_{intra} = E_{bond} + E_{angle} + E_{torsion} + E_{oop}$

Solvation free energy

Polar solvation
free energy
G_{elec} (GBMV)

Non-polar solvation
free energy
$G_{np} = \gamma \times SASA + b$

Solute Entropy
Constant

Figure 3.
Calculation of binding energy using the MM-GB/SA approach [36].

where ΔG_{bind} shows the free energy of ligand-protein total binding; ΔE_{MM} reflects the total gas phase energy (sum of $\Delta E_{internal}$, $\Delta E_{electrostatic}$, and ΔE_{vdw}); ΔG_{sol} is the sum of polar ($\Delta G_{PB/GB}$) and non-polar (ΔG_{SA}) contributions to solvation; and $-T\Delta S$ refers to the conformational binding entropy (commonly calculated by normal-mode analysis). $\Delta E_{internal}$ shows the internal energy that arises from different bond, angle, and dihedral in molecular mechanics (MM) force field (in the MM/PBSA and MM/GBSA, this always amounts to zero as shown in single trajectory of a complex calculation). $\Delta E_{electrostatic}$ and ΔE_{vdw} are the electrostatic and van der Waals energies resulted from the calculation of MM, while $\Delta G_{PB/GB}$ shows the polar contribution to the solvation free energy (calculated using Poisson–Boltzmann (PB) or generalized Born (GB) method). ΔG_{SA} is the nonpolar solvation free energy that is usually computed using a linear function of the solvent-accessible surface area (SASA). E_{MM} is molecular mechanical energy calculated from CHARMM force field, G_{elec} and G_{NP} are electrostatic polar components and non-solvation free energy. TS term refers to the entropy of the solute which is assumed to be constant between one set of poses for the same ligand on the active side. E_{MM} is a gas phase forcefield energy and consists of internal energy (E_{int}), electrostatic energy (E_{elec}) and van der Waals energy components. E_{int} is further divided into E_{bond}, E_{angle}, $E_{torsion}$ and E_{oop} to calculate account energy related to bonds, angles, torque and outside as shown in **Figure 3**.

MM/GBSA and MM/PBSA have been successfully applied to predict the binding free energies for various ligand sesquiterpenoid/sesquiterpenoid alcohol to protein COX-1/COX-2, but the previous studies mostly focused on certain specific systems and the prediction results cannot afford the overall accuracy of MM/PBSA and MM/GBSA for ligand-protein systems.

3. Ligand sesquiterpenoid

Ligand sequiterpenoid was obtained from pubchem.ncbi.nlm.nih.gov, such as (alpha-bulnesene (CID94275), alpha-guaiene (CID107152), and seychellene (CID519743). Also, sesquiterpenoid alcohols, including alpha-Patchouli alcohol isomers (CID442384, CID521903, CID6432585, CID3080622, CID10955174, and CID56928117) as 3D-SDF format. Then, its energy was minimized which files were converted to 3D-PDB format by Open Babel 2.3.1 in Hex 8.0 as the ligands prepared for virtual screening [6, 8, 11, 31]. The structures of studied ligands are shown in **Figure 4**.

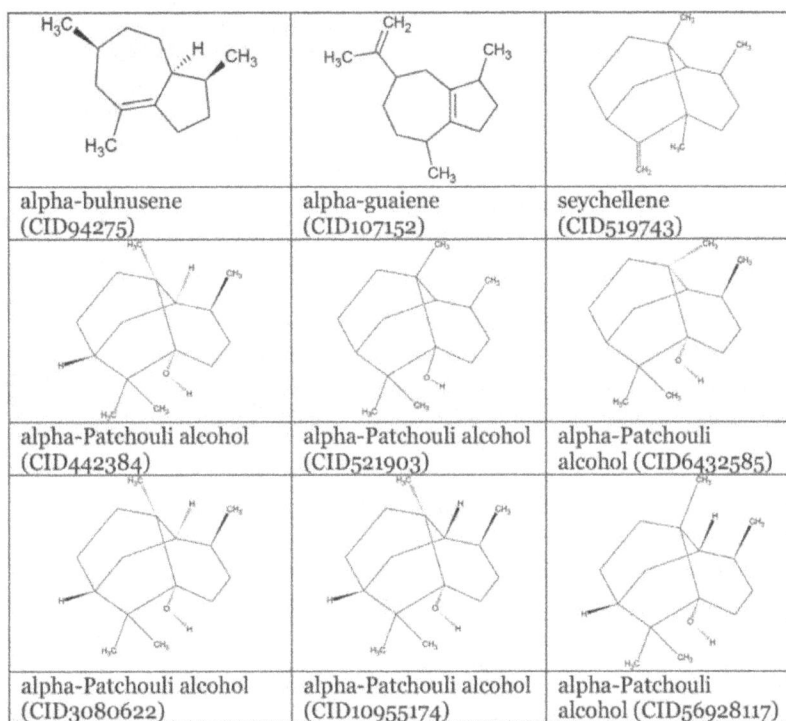

Figure 4.
Structure of sequiterpenoid and sesquiterpenoid alcohols Pogostemon herba.

Sesquiterpenoid, such as alpha-bulnesene (CID94275), alpha-guaiene (CID107152), and seychellene (CID519743) has molecular weight 204.35 g/mol, molecular formula $C_{15}H_{24}$, and XLogP3-AA: 4.60; 4.6; and 5.10 respectively (**Table 1**). And alpha-patchouli alcohol isomers has molecular weight: 222.36634 g/mol; molecular formula:

$C_{15}H_{26}O$; XLogP3-AA: 4.1; H-Bond Donor: 1; and H-Bond Acceptor: 1. The number of isomers of alpha-Patchouli alcohol is six. In **Figure 4**

Description	sequiterpenoid			sesquiterpenoid alcohol
	CID94275	CID107152	CID519743	CID442384, CID521903, CID6432585, CID3080622, CID1095517,CID56928117
Molecular Weight (g mol^{-1})	204.35	204.35	204.35	222.36
Kinase inhibitor	−1.33	−1.33	−1.30	−0.88
Nuclear receptor inhibitor	0.19	0.19	0.27	0.55
Protease inhibitor	−0.60	−0.60	−0.50	−0.32
Enzyme inhibitor	0.07	0.07	0.28	0.40
xlogP3-AA	4.6	4.60	5.10	4.10
H-Bond donor	0	0	0	1
H-Bond aseptor	0	0	0	1

Table 1.
Physical–chemical properties and predicted activity of sesquiterpenoids and sequiterpenoid alcohols Pogostemon herba.

2D-sesquiterpernoid/sesquiterpenoid alcohol, such as alpha-bulnesene (CID94275), alpha-guaiene, and seychellene (CID519743), and alpha-Patchouli isomers (CID442384, CID521903, CID6432585, CID3080622, CID10955174, and CID56928117) show the different position of hydroxyl group and hydrogen atom. The 3D structure of sesquiterpenoid/sesquiterpenoid alcohol was retrieved in 3D-SDF format from http://pubchem.ncbi.nlm.nih.gov/. For the preparation of docking, 3D-SDF format of isomers was converted to 3D-PDB using open babel software. This program helps to search, convert, analyze, or store data which has a wide range of applications in the different fields of molecular modeling, computational chemistry, and so forth. For a common user, it helps to apply chemistry aspects without worrying about the low level details of chemical information. It also converts crystallographic file formats (CIF, ShelX), reaction formats (MDLRXN), molecular dynamics and docking (AutoDock, Amber), 3D viewers (Chem3D, Molden), and chemical kinetics and thermodynamics (ChemKin, Termo) [6, 8].

4. Cyclooxygenase protein receptor (COX-1 and COX-2)

3D model from PDB ID: 1PTH was obtained from SWISS-MODEL repository for cyclooxygenase-1 (COX-1) (http://www.rcsb.org/pdb/explore/explore.do?structure Id=1pth) and 3D model from PDB ID: 6COX for cyclooxygenase-2 (COX-2) [6, 8]. We used Ramachandran plot analysis for validation protein receptor [32].

In **Figure 5** shows the Ramachandran plot analysis of COX-1 and COX-2 protein receptor before rigid docking. It showed that COX-1 protein receptor had 97.5% favored regions, 2.4% allowed regions, and, 0.2% outlier regions. Whereas, COX-2 protein receptor had 81.9% favored regions, 15.4% allowed regions and 2.7% outlier regions. Ramachandran plot displays the main chain torsion angles phi, psi (φ, Ψ) (Ramachandran angles) in a protein of known structure. The model was verified to guarantee the validity of programming and algorithms implemented. Results of the validity test showed that amino acid residues were distributed at the most favorable region in the Ramachandran plot. This is an indication of the stereochemical quality

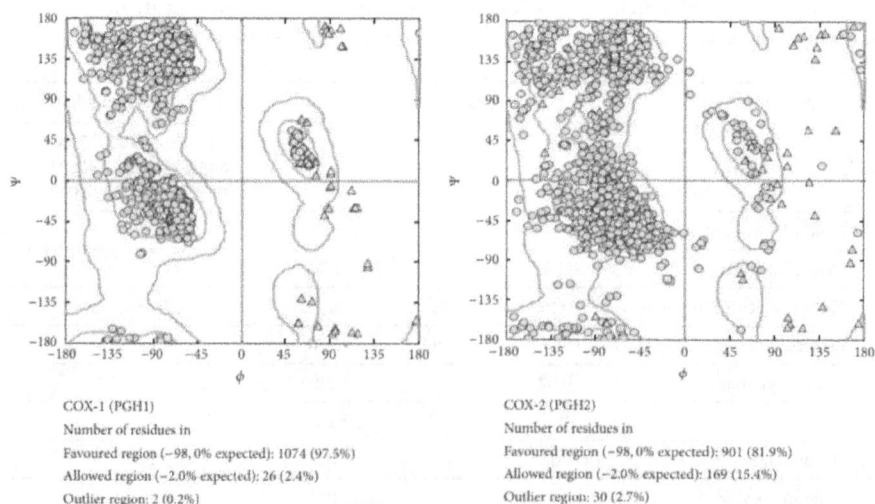

COX-1 (PGH1)

Number of residues in

Favoured region (−98, 0% expected): 1074 (97.5%)

Allowed region (−2.0% expected): 26 (2.4%)

Outlier region: 2 (0.2%)

COX-2 (PGH2)

Number of residues in

Favoured region (−98, 0% expected): 901 (81.9%)

Allowed region (−2.0% expected): 169 (15.4%)

Outlier region: 30 (2.7%)

Figure 5.
Ramachandran plot analysis of COX-1 and COX-2.

of the model taken for the structural analysis and also validated the target-ligand binding efficacy of the structure. The Ramachandran plot presents the angle of phi-psi torsion of all residues in the structure (except those at the chain termini) which were classified according to their regions in the quadrangle. The most favored regions are colored yellow, additional allowed/generously allowed region, and outlier regions are indicated as blue and pink fields, respectively [6, 8, 32].

5. Molecular docking ligand and binding energy interaction sesquiterpenoid/sesquiterpenoid alcohols to protein COX-1 and COX-2

We used Hex8.0 software (http://hex.loria.fr) for rigid docking to compute possible interaction COX-1 and COX-2 with (alpha-bulnesene (CID94275), alpha-guaiene (CID107152), seychellene (CID519743) and sesquiterpenoid alcohols such as alpha-Patchouli alcohol isomers (CID442384, CID521903, CID6432585, CID3080622, CID10955174, and CID56928117) on the interaction site. Output of the docking was refined using Discovery Studio Client 3.5 software. We used Discovery Studio Client 3.5 to perform interactions, ligand binds to COX-1/COX-2 and Ramachandran plot analysis.

The repeat rigid docking used Hex 8.0 software to compute possible interaction COX-1 and COX-2 with sesquiterpenoid/sesquiterpenoid alcohols such as alpha-bulnesene (CID94275), alpha-guaiene, seychellene (CID519743), and alpha-patchouli alcohol isomers (CID442384, CID521903, CID6432585, CID3080622, CID10955174, and CID56928117) on its interaction site and the data are represented by Discovery Studio 3.5 software in (**Figure 5(a1–l1)**). The interaction site position of COX-1/COX-2-sesquiterpenoid/sesquiterpenoid alcohol complexes were analyzed using Discovery Studio-3.5 Client software to get the receptor-ligand interaction and Ramachandran plot, as shown in Figure 5; some of them are alpha-patchouli alcohol isomers-COX-1/COX-2 complexes.

In **Table 2** and **Figure 6**, the interactions active site of ligand sesquiterpenoid/ sesquiterpenoid alcohol with COX-1 and COX-2 protein receptor showed the differences in the position active site. The different positions were analyzed and presented in the Ramachandran plot analysis and its amino acid residues in the receptor active site of COX-1 and COX-2 in which hydrogen atoms and hydroxyl groups on each of the 3D-isomers of alpha-patchouli alcohol structure were in different position (**Figure 4**). The results of docking and analysis of the active site also show that all ligands sesquiterpenoid/sesquiterpenoid alcohol are in the catalytic domain. Thus, all the compounds have the capability of blocking oxygenated reaction and reaction peroxides; currently substrate arachidonic acid becomes PGH2.

Each ligand, CID521903, was seen interacting with HEM682B group in COX-2-CID521903 complexes. This result proved that it would lead to inhibition of enzymatic reactions occurring COX-1 and COX-2. The analysis of active site showed that there are any difference and similarities of the active site of all ligand alpha-patchouli alcohol isomers which is interact with receptor proteins COX-1 and COX-2. This difference is caused by different stereoisomers of hydrogen atoms and hydroxyl group in alpha-patchouli alcohol isomers. The different position active site the complexes have led to interaction types, such as hydrogen bond, van der Waals, electrostatic and covalent bond. The different types of interactions in this complex will certainly affect its binding free energy.

No.	Virtual modeling	Amino acid residues in the active site (by Hex 8.0 software and then Discovery Studio 3.5 software)	
		COX-1	COX-2
1.	alpha-Patchouli alcohol CID442384	TRP141A, GLU142A, SER145A, ASN146A, LEU226B, GLY227B, ASP231B, GLN243B, GLY237B, ASN239B, LEU240B, ASP238B, ARG335B	TRP139A, GLU140A, SER143A, ASN144A, LEU145A, GLY235B, GLU236B, THR237B, LEU238B, GLN241B, GLN330B
2.	alpha-Patchouli alcohol CID521903	SER123A, ASN124A, LEU125A, ILE126A, PRO127A, SER128A, PRO129A, GLN372A, PHE373A, GLN274A, LYS534A, PRO544B, GLU545B	LYS211B, THR212B, ASP213B, HIS214B, LYS215B, ARG222B, ILE274B, GLN298B, GLU290B, VAL291B, HEM682B
3.	alpha-Patchouli alcohol CID643285	TRP141A, GLU142A, SER145A, ASN146A, LEU226B, ASP231B, GLY237B, ASP238B, ASN239B, LEU240B, GLN243B, ARG335B	TRP139A, GLU140A, SER143A, ASN144A, LEU145A, THR237B, LEU238B, GLY235B, GLU236B, GLN241B, GLN330B, LYS333B
4.	alpha-Patchouli alcohol CID3080622	SER123A, ASN124A, ILE126A, PRO127A, SER128A, PRO129A, GLN372A, PHE373A, GLN374A, LYS534A, PRO544B, GLU545B	TRP139A, SER143A, ASN144A, LEU145A, GLY235B, GLU236B, THR237B, LEU238B, GLN241B, LYS333B
5.	alpha-Patchouli alcohol CID10955174	TRP141A, GLU142A, SER145A, ASN146A, LEU226B, ASP231B, GLY237B, ASP238B, ASN239B, LEU240B, GLN243B, ARG335B	TRP139A, GLU140A, SER143A, ASN144A, LEU145A, GLY235B, GLU236B, THR237B, LEU238B, GLN241B, GLN330B, LYS33B
6.	alpha-Patchouli alcohol CID56928117	Electrostatic: ASN146B. Van der Walls: LEU226A, GLY237A, ASP238A, ASN239A, LEU240A, GLU241A, GLN243A, ARG335A, TRP141B, GLU142B, SER145B	Electrostatic: SER143B. Van der Walls: GLY235A, GLU236A, THR237A, LEU238A, ASP239A, GLN241A, LYS333A, TRP139B, GLU140B, ASN144B, LEU145B
7.	alpha-bulnesene CID94275	Van der Walls: VAL147A, LYS224A, ALA225A, LEU226A, GLY227A, ASP231A, GLY233A, GLY237A, ASP238A, ASN239A, LEU240A, ARG335A, TRP141B, GLU142B, SER145B, ASN146B, VAL147B	Van der Walls: GLY225A, ASP229A, GLY235A, GLU236A, LEU238A, GLN241A, GLN330A, THR237A, LYS333A, SER143B, TRP139B, GLU140B, ASN144B, LEU145B
8.	alpha-guaiene CID107152	Van der Walls: TRP141A, GLU142A, SER145A, ASN146A, LEU226B, GLY227B, ASP231B, GLY237B, ASN239B, ASP238B, LEU240B, GLU241B, GLN243B, ARG335B	Van der Walls: GLY225A, ASP229A, ASN231A, GLY235A, GLU236A, THR237A, GLN241A, GLN330A, LYS333A, TRP139B, GLU140B, SER143B, ASN144B, LEU145B, LEU238A
9.	Seychellene CID519743	Van der Walls: PRO544A, GLU545A, SER123B, ASN124B, LEU125B, ILE126B, PRO127B, SER128B, PHE373B, GLN372B, GLN374B, LYS534B	Van der Walls: ASP213A, HIS214A, LYS215A, LYS211A, THR212A, ARG222A, ILE274A, GLN289A, GLU290A, VAL291A, HEM682A

Table 2.
Analysis of virtual modeling of COX-1/COX-2-sesquiterpenoid/sesquiterpenoid alcohol complexes.

6. Molecular dynamic screening of sesquiterpenoid/sesquiterpenoid alcohol *Pogostemon herba* as predicted cyclooxygenase inhibitor selective

After the results of the rigid docking to compute possible interaction COX-1 and COX-2 with (alpha-bulnesene (CID94275), alpha-guaiene (CID107152), and

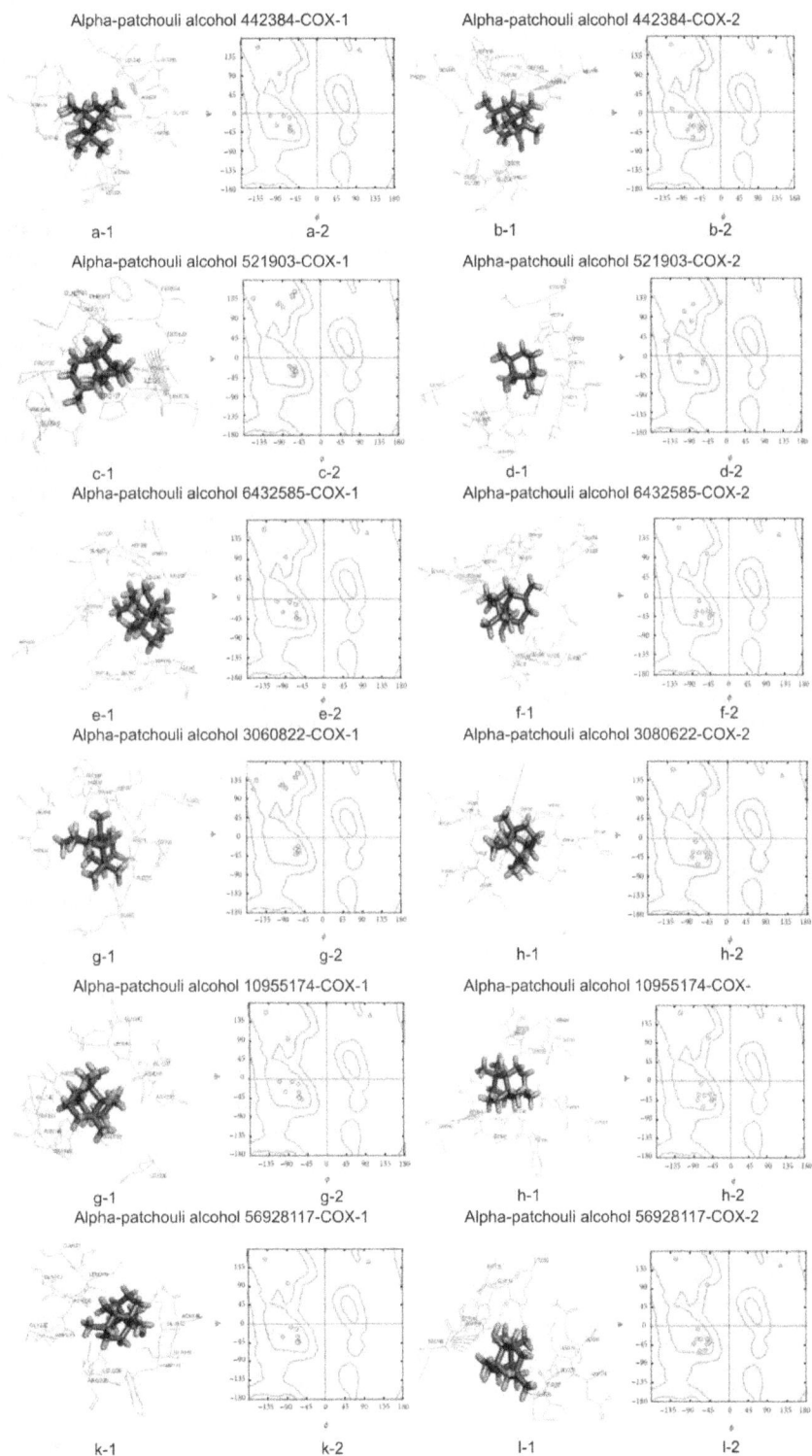

Figure 6.
Modeling analysis alpha-patchouli alcohol isomer in complex with COX-1 and COX-2. (a1) – (l1) 3D active site structure of COX-1/COX-2-alpha-patchouli alcohol isomers complexes; (a2) to (l2) Ramachandran plot analysis of COX-1/COX-2-alpha-patchouli alcohol complexes using discovery studio 3.5 viewer Software.

seychellene (CID519743). And also, sesquiterpenoid alcohol, such as alpha-Patchouli alcohol isomers (CID442384, CID521903, CID6432585, CID3080622, CID10955174, and CID56928117) to performed active visualization-interaction 2D and 3D, and binding energy using Discovery Studio 3.5 software. The output of the docking, visualization, and binding energy calculation using AMBER12 software and Virtual Molecular Dynamics 1.9.1 obtained the most possible native complex structure of sesquiterpenoid/sesquiterpenoid alcohol of CID94275, CID107152, CID519743, CID442384, CID521903, CID6432585, CID3080622, CID10955174, and CID56928117, respectively, that bind with COX-1 and COX-2 in molecular dynamic with Model Solvent of MM-PBSA (Molecular Mechanics Poisson-Boltzmann Surface Area), which included both backbone and side-chains movements. Therefore, we used AMBER12 to refine the candidate models according to a binding energy calculation for scoring of virtual screening sesquiterpenoid/sesquiterpenoid alcohol compounds as selective inhibitor for COX-1 and/or COX-2. Molecular dynamics (MD) were carried out using AMBER12 and the AMBER-99 force field. The initial structure of the sesquiterpenoid/sesquiterpenoid alcohol inhibitor complex was taken for each compound from the Hex 8.0 docking study. The ligand force fields parameters were taken from the General Amber force Field (GAFF), whereas AM1 ESP atomic partial charges were assigned to the inhibitors. Prior to the free MD simulations, two steps of relaxation were carried out; in the first step, we kept the protein fixed with a constraint of 500 Kcal·mol^{-1} · °A^{-1}. In the second step, the inhibitor structures were relaxed for 0.5 pico second, during which the protein atoms were restrained to the X-ray coordinates with a force constant of 500 Kcal·mol^{-1} · °A^{-1}. In the final step, all restraints were removed and the complexes were relaxed for 1 pico second. The temperature of the relaxed system was then equilibrated at 300 Kelvin through 20 pico second of MD using 2 fs time steps. A constant volume periodic boundary was set to equilibrate the temperature of the system by the Langevin dynamics using a collision frequency of 10 ps^{-1} and a velocity limit of five temperature units. During the temperature equilibration routine, the complex in the solvent box was restrained to the initial coordinates with a weak force constant of 10 Kcal·mol^{-1} · °A^{-1}. The final coordinates of the temperature equilibration routine (after 20 ps) were then used to complete a 1 ns molecular dynamics routine using 2 fs time steps, during which the temperature was kept at 300 Kelvin. For the Langevin dynamics a collision frequency of 1 ps^{-1} and a velocity limit of 20 temperature units were used. The pressure of the solvated system was equilibrated at 1 bar at a certain density in a constant pressure periodic boundary by an isotropic pressure scaling method employing a pressure relaxation time of 2 ps. The time step of the free MD simulations was 2 fs with a cut-off of 9°A for the non-bonded interaction, and SHAKE was employed to keep all bonds involving hydrogen atoms rigid. Calculation of binding energy was administered using this equation:

$$\Delta G_{bind} = G_{complex} - \left[G_{protein} + G_{ligand} \right]$$

[6, 8, 33–37].

We were using AMBER12 software and Virtual Molecular Dynamics 1.9.1 to simulate the most possible native complex structure of sesquiterpenoid/sesquiterpenoid alcohol (CID94275, CID107152, CID519743, CID442384, CID521903, CID6432585, CID3080622, CID10955174, and CID56928117), respectively, that binds with COX-1 and COX-2 in molecular dynamic with MM-PBSA Model Solvent. The MD simulations of the sesquiterpenoid/sesquiterpenoid alcohol-inhibitor, some of them are alpha-patchouli alcohol-COX-1/COX-2 complexes. The structure of the complexes is shown in **Figure 7(a–f)** and **(j–o)**. We also acquire the results of the analysis of 200 poses: the complex energy, energy ligand protein, and energy. The binding energy was calculated use the following equation:

$$\Delta G_{bind} = G_{complex} - [G_{protein} + G_{ligand}]$$

as shown in **Figure 7(g–i)**, **(p–r)** and **(o)**.

Analysis of the active site and the binding energies COX-1/COX-2-sesquiterpenoid/sesquiterpenoid alcohol are by Discovery Studio 3.5 and Amber 12, summarized and presented in **Figure 7** (s).

The different position active site the complexes have led to interaction types, such as hydrogen bond, van der Waals, electrostatic and covalent bond. The different types of interactions in this complex will certainly affect its binding free energy. The use of Poisson-Boltzmann (PB) and Generalized Born (GB) characterized the binding free energy calculation model solvent MMPB/SA and MM-GB/SA in computing the electrostatic component of the solvation free energy. The following equation was employed in binding free energy of the protein-ligand complex.

$$\Delta G = \Delta H - T\Delta S \qquad (8)$$

T is the temperature of the system at 300 Kelvin. The free binding energy (ΔG_{binds}) of the protein-ligand-complex were evaluated using MMPBSA (Molecular Mechanics Poison Blotzmann Surface Area) method as implemented in Discovery Studio 3.5 and AMBER12. MMPBSA has always been considered as a proper method to compare binding energies of similar ligands. MMPBSA measures the binding free energy based on thermodynamic cycle in which molecular mechanical energy and the continuum solvent approaches are simultaneously used [6, 8, 33, 38]. The calculation of binding free energy is computed as:

$$\Delta G_{bind} = G_{complex} - [G_{protein} + G_{ligand}] \qquad (9)$$

In (5.2), $G_{complex}$ is the absolute free energy of the complex, $G_{protein}$ is the absolute free energy of the protein, and G_{ligand} is the absolute free energy of the ligand [6, 8, 33, 38]. The free energy of each term was estimated as a sum of the three terms:

$$[G] = [E_{MM}] + [G_{sol}] - T \cdot [S] \qquad (10)$$

$[G_{MM}]$ is the molecular mechanics energy of the molecule expressed as the sum of the internal energy (bond, angle, and dihedral) (E_{int}), electrostatic energy (E_{ele}), and van der Waals term (E_{vdw}):

$$[E_{MM}] = [E_{int}] + [E_{ele}] + [E_{vdw}] \qquad (11)$$

$[E_{ele}]$ solvation energy can be categorized as polar and nonpolar part. Polar part gives electrostatic contribution to solvation by solving the linear Poisson Boltzmann equation within the solvent's continuum model [33]. The binding energy calculation in AMBER12 includes preparation, minimization, heating, and energy calculations (complex, protein, and ligand). We extracted 200 snapshots (at time intervals of 2 ps) for each species (complex, protein, and ligand). Furthermore, the visualization using virtual model dynamic (VMD 1.9.1 software) is shown in **Figure 7(a–f)** and **(j–o)**, and then the binding energy calculation can be obtained from the data ligand energy, protein energy, and energy complex by AMBER12, 200 times/poses, respectively; next, the binding free energy calculation is calculated by Eq. (7.2) and shown in **Figure 7(g)**, **(h)**, **(i)**, **(p)**, **(q)**, and **(r)** and summarized in **Figure 5(s)**. **Figure 5(s)** shows that the binding energy calculation (PBSA Model

Solvent) of COX-1 CID442384 complexes (-28.386 ± 1.102 Kcal/mol) was smaller than the COX-2 CID442384 complexes (-16.215 ± 0.985 Kcal/mol) and also ligands CID6432585, CID3080622, CID10955174, and CID56928117. The similar research, docking studies ligand salicin compound from D. gangeticum to COX-1 and COX-2 protein receptor, showed high binding affinity COX-2 protein (-5 Kcal/mol) and lesser interaction with COX-1 (-3.79 Kcal/mol). Therefore, salicin could predict as COX-2 inhibitor selective and anti-cancerous compound [6].

E_{binds} (ΔG) was determined on the basis of calculation of the Eq. (5.2). Gligand value is influenced by the type of ligand. Gligand will affect the value Ebinds and ratio of E_{binds} COX-1 and E_{binds} COX-2. Hence, in-silico analysis can be used as an approach to determine the selectivity of the ligand as an inhibitor of COX-1/COX-2. Ebinds (binding energy calculations) seychellene (CID519743) (**Figure 7(s)**) showed as candidate non-selective COX inhibitor and it's similar to value of selective IC$_{50}$, as shown in **Figure 8**.

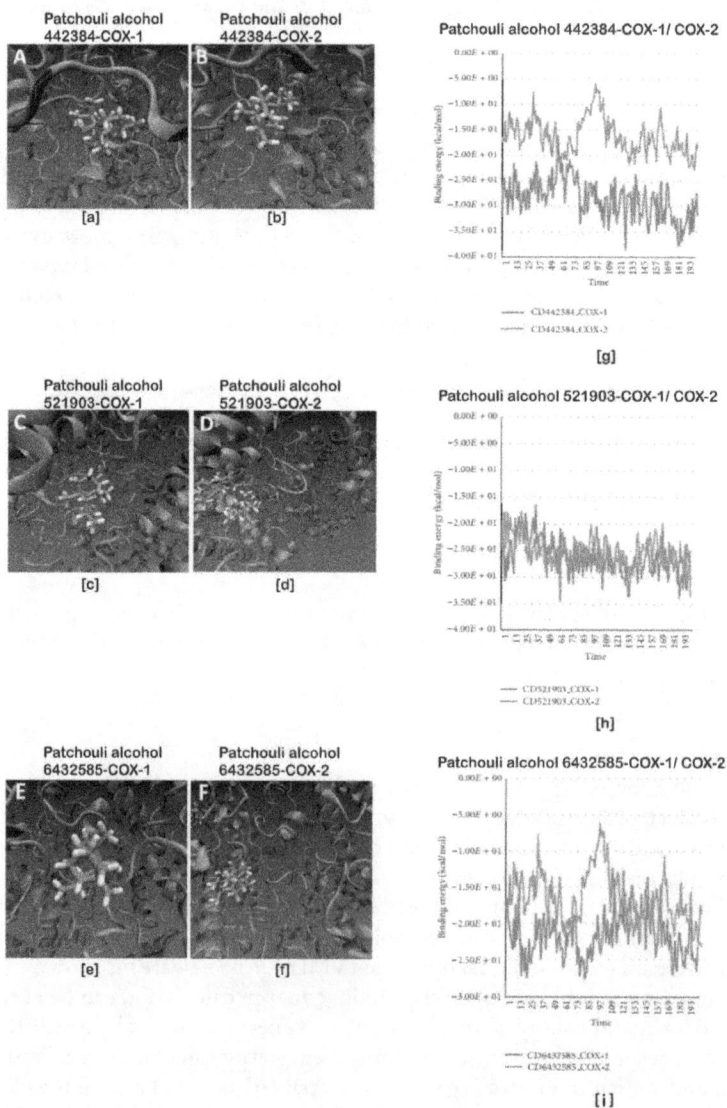

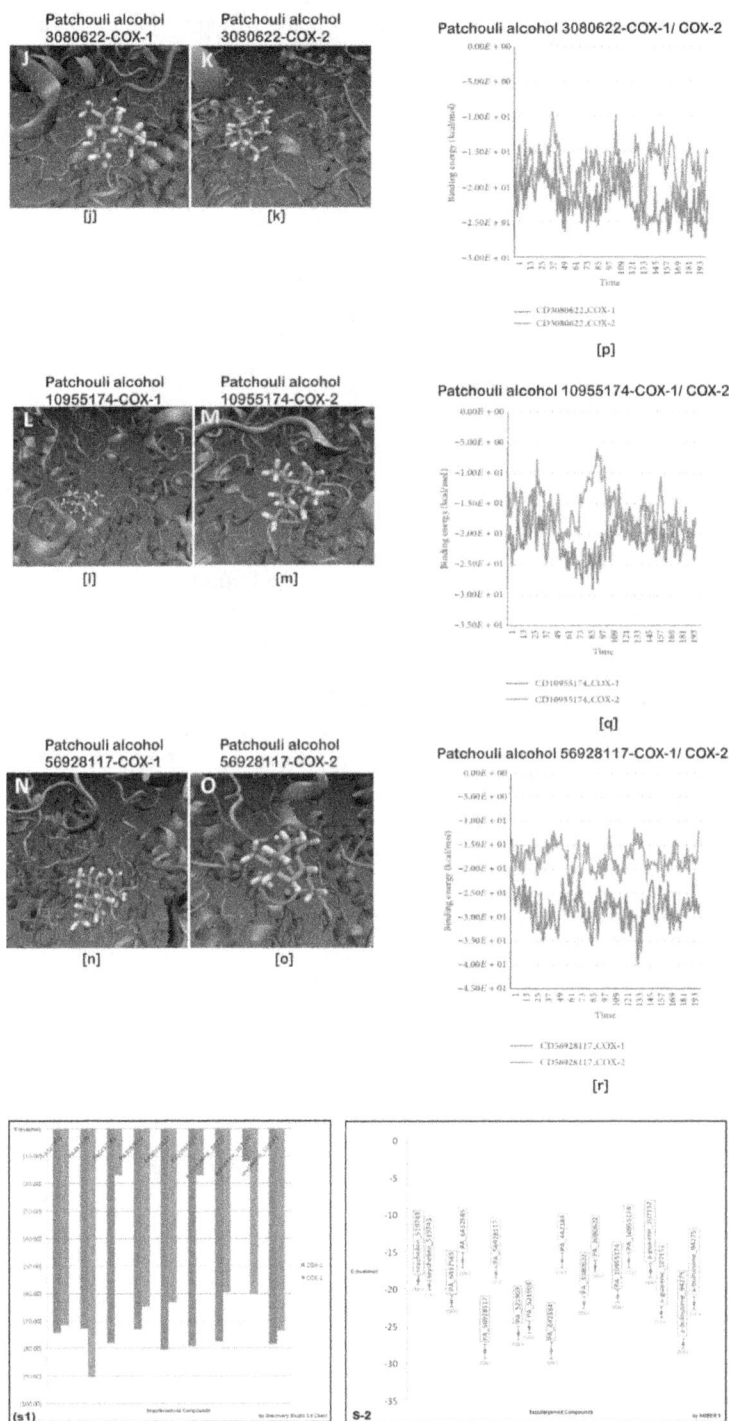

Figure 7.
Binding energy calculation of alpha-patchouli alcohol isomers binds to COX-1/COX-2. (a) and (f) and (j)–(o) virtual molecule dynamic complexes of COX-1/COX-2-alpha-patchouli alcohol isomers. (g), (h), (i), (p),(q), and (r) comparison of binding energy calculation of alpha-patchouli alcohol isomer-COX-1 (blue) and COX-2 (red) complexes. (s) Histogram of binding energy calculation of COX-1 (blue)/COX-2 (red) sesquiterpenoid/sesquiterpenoid alcohol complexes by discovery studio 3.5 (s-1) and Amber 12 (s-2).

The relationship binding energy, K_i and IC_{50} is defined by Eq. (5.5) and (5.6) [39, 40].

$$\Delta G_{bind} = 2.303 \, R \cdot T \log K_i \tag{12}$$

$$\text{For competitive inhibition}: K_i = (IC_{50} - E/2)/(S/Km + 1)$$

$$\text{For uncompetitive inhibition}: K_i = (IC_{50} - E/2)/(Km/S + 1)$$

$$\text{if } S = Km, K_i = IC_{50}/2;$$

$$\text{if } S >> K_m, K_i << IC_{50};$$

$$\text{if } S << K_m \, K_i \approx IC_{50}.$$

For non-competitive inhibition: $K_i = IC_{50}$ when $S = K_m$ or $S << K_m$ and for tightly bound inhibitor:

$$K_i = IC_{50} - E/2 \tag{13}$$

where: E = enzyme, S = Substrate, P=Product.

The latest development is more selective selective COX-2 drugs, such as valdecoxib (Bextra™) and etoricoxib (Arcoxi™) and lumiracoxib (Prexige). Several COX-2-selective drugs in NSAIDs are presented in **Figure 9**. The classification of COX inhibition is based on the potential inhibition of COX isoforms and specifically the IC_{50} ratio of COX-1 and COX-2 (or selectivity index) [20].

Eq. (5.5) can be used as the COX-1/COX-2 selectivity approach in in-silico analysis, which without calculating for competitive, un-competitive and non-competitive, shows that ΔG_{bind} are directly proportional to IC50 values.

While the selectivity of COX-1/COX-2 is expressed in the equation:

$$IC_{50} \text{ selectivity, } COX - 1/COX - 2 = \log \, (IC_{50}, \text{ratio } (COX - 2/COX - 1)) \tag{14}$$

Therefore selectivity in in-silico analysis can be expressed as:

$$E_{bind} \text{ selectivity, } COX - 1/COX - 2 = \log \, (E_{bind}, \text{ratio } (COX - 2/COX - 1)) \tag{15}$$

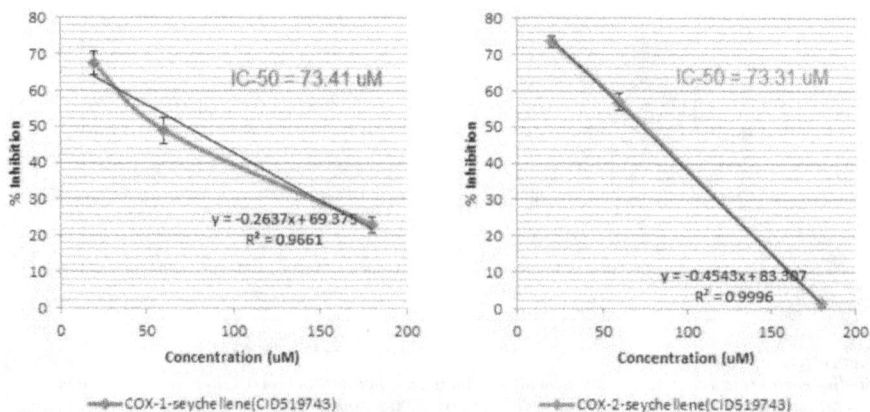

Figure 8.
Regression linier analyses of IC_{50} fraction-5 to COX-1 and COX-2 [39].

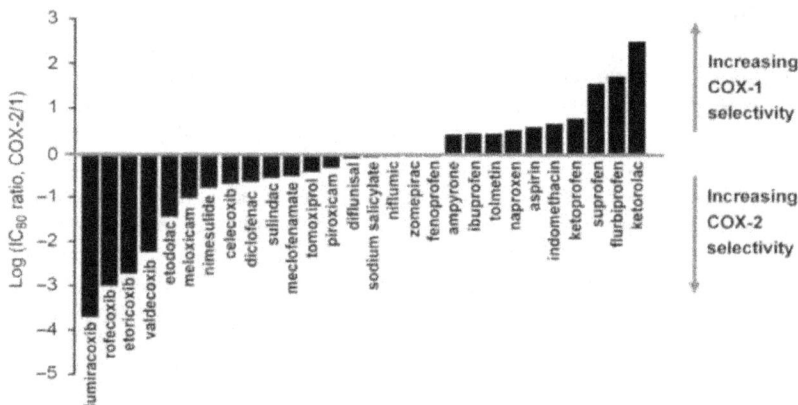

Figure 9.
The relative selectivity of COX-1 and COX-2 inhibitors based on the IC_{80} ratio is declared logarithmic, so 0 is the baseline, that is, the compound in the line is equiactive to COX-1 and COX-2. Compounds above the COX-1-selective line and below are COX-2 selective [34].

According Eq. (5.5), selectivities Ebinds and selectivities IC50 some of them are complexes of CID442384, CID519743, CID3060622, CID107152, and CID94275 with COX-1/COX-2, as shown in **Figure 10**.

Collectively, our results suggest that alpha-Patchouli alcohol (CID442384) as candidate COX-2 inhibitor selective, alpha-guaiene (CID107152), alpha bulnesene (CID94275), alpha patchouli alcohol isomers (CID3060622, CID6432585, CID10955174, and CID56928117) as candidate COX-1 inhibitor selective, and alpha-patchouli alcohol CID521903, seychellene as candidate COX non selective. These in silico analysis data will be completed with the biological activity analysis.

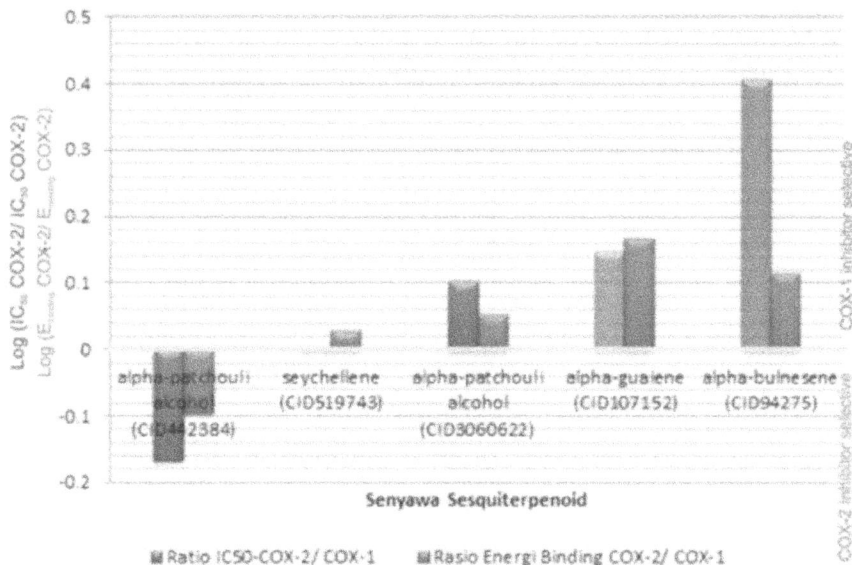

Figure 10.
Selectivities of IC_{50} versus E_{binds} sesquiterpenoid/sesquiterpenoid alcohol Pogostemon herba *to COX-1/COX-2.*

7. Conclusion

Exploration of sesquiterpenoid/sesquiterpenoid alcohol compounds as inhibitors of COX isoenzymes as development of group NSAIDs, was carried out by means of in silico tools. The binding energy calculation (using PBSA Model Solvent) of sesquiterpenoid/sesquiterpenoid alcohol compounds: alpha patchouli alcohol (CID521903) and seychellene (CID519743) were identified as the candidates of non-selective inhibitor; alpha bulnesene (CID94275), alpha guaiene (CID107152), and alpha-patchouli alcohol isomers (CID6432585, CID3080622, CID10955174, while CID56928117) had been suggested as the candidate for a selective COX-1 inhibitor. Whereas, alpha-patchouli alcohol (CID442384) was the candidate for a selective COX-2 inhibitor.

Acknowledgments

This study was supported by Doctoral program scholarship of "Sandwich-Like Program 2013," DGHE, Ministry of Education and Culture, RI. The authors acknowledge all facilities of Bioinformatics Laboratory Department of Creation Core, Ritsumeikan University, for providing the in silico analyses. Special thanks are due to Prof. Takhesi Kikuchi (my sensei), Masanari Matsuoka, Antonius Christianto, Michirou Kabata, Sayaka Ohara, Yousuke Kawai, and working group Bioinformatic Laboratory, Biwako Kutsasu Campus, Ritsumeikan University, for helpful support analysis and discussions. And also my wife (Sri Wahjoeni), my son (Damara Setyowijayanto Raharjo), Prof. Fatchiyah, Prof. Chanif Mahdi, Prof. Sutiman, Dr. Nurdiana, Lectures of Biology Dept. Brawijaya University, Lectures Academic of Pharmacy and Food Analysis "Putra Indonesia Malang", Yayasan Putera Indonesia Malang, and Pharmacy Dept. Faculty Medicine Brawijaya University.

Conflict of interests

The authors declare no conflict of interests.

Author details

Sentot Joko Raharjo
Academic of Pharmacy and Food Analysis "Putra Indonesia Malang", Malang,
Indonesia

*Address all correspondence to: sjraharjo.akafarma@pimedu.ac.id;
sjraharjo03@gmail.com

IntechOpen

References

[1] Ge H, Wang Y, Li C, Chen N, Xie Y, Xu M. Molecular dynamics-based virtual screening: Accelerating drug discovery process by high performance computing. Journal of Chemical Information and Modeling. 2013; 53(10):2757-2764. DOI: 10.1021/ ci400391s

[2] Durikovic R and Motooka T. Molecular dynamics simulation and visualization. In Proceedings of the International Conference on Information Visualisation 1999; 16 July 1999; London, England: IEEE; 1999. pp. 334-339

[3] Jeanmonod DJ, Rebecca, Suzuki K, et al. Protein-protein and protein-ligand docking. London, United Kingdom: Intech Open; 2018. pp. 64-81. DOI: 10.5772/56376

[4] Verma R. In silico studies of small molecule interactions with enzymes reveal aspects of catalytic function. Catalysts. 2017;7(212):1-26. DOI: 10.3390/catal7070212

[5] Reddy AS, Pati SP, Kumar PP, Pradeep HN, Sastry GN. Virtual screening in drug discovery—a computational perspective. Current Protein and Peptide Science. 2007;8: 329-351. DOI: 10.2174/1389203077 81369427

[6] Raharjo SJ, Mahdi C, Nurdiana N, Kikuchi T, Fatchiyah F. Binding energy calculation of patchouli alcohol isomer cyclooxygenase complexes suggested as COX-1/COX-2 selective inhibitor. Advances in Bioinformatics. 2014;2014: 1-12. DOI: 10.1155/2014/850628

[7] Ghalami-Choobar B, Moghadam H. Molecular docking based on virtual screening, molecular dynamics and atoms in molecules studies to identify the potential human epidermal receptor

2 intracellular domain inhibitors. Physics Chemistry Research. 2018;6(1): 83-103. DOI: 10.22036/pcr.2017.88200. 1385

[8] Raharjo SJ, Kikuchi T. Molecular dynamic screening sesquiterpenoid pogostemon herba as suggested cyclooxygenase inhibitor. Acta Information Medical. 2016;24(5):332-337. DOI: 10.5455/aim.2016.24.332-337

[9] Raharjo SJ. In silico and in vitro analyses α- and γ-guaiene Pogostemon herbs for cyclooxygenase isoenzyme inhibitor. In Proceeding Int. Conf. Essent. Oil; 11–12 October 2017; Malang —Indonesia; 2017;1(1):56-65

[10] Raharjo SJ, Fatchiyah F. Virtual screening of compounds from the patchouli oil of *Pogostemon* herba for COX-1 inhibition. Bioinformation. 2013; 9(6):321-324. DOI: 10.6026/ 97320630009321

[11] Raharjo SJ, Mahdi C, Nurdiana N, Nellen W, Fatchiyah F. Patchouli alcohol isomers *Pogostemon* herba predicted virtually. Journal of Biological Research. 2014;18(2):98-101

[12] Kastritis PL, Bonvin AMJJ. Are scoring functions in protein-protein docking ready to predict interactomes? Clues from a novel binding affinity benchmark. Journal of Proteome Research. 2010;9(5):2216-2225. DOI: 10.1021/pr9009854

[13] Hou T, Wang J, Li Y, Wang W. Assessing the performance of the MM/ PBSA and MM/GBSA methods. Journal of Chemical Information and Modeling. 2011;51:69-82. DOI: 10.1021/ci100275a

[14] Wang J, Hou T, Xu X. Recent advances in free energy calculations with a combination of molecular mechanics and continuum models.

Current Computer-Aided Drug Design. 2006;**2**(3):287-306. DOI: 10.2174/157340906778226454

[15] Gohlke H, Klebe G. Approaches to the description and prediction of the binding affinity of small-molecule ligands to macromolecular receptors. Angewandte Chemie, International Edition. 2002;**41**(55): 2644-2676. DOI: 10.1002/1521-3773 (20020802)41:15<2644::AID-ANIE2644>3.0.CO;2-O

[16] Bissantz C, Kuhn B, Stahl M. A medicinal chemist's guide to molecular interactions. Journal of Medicinal Chemistry. 2010;**53**(14):5061-5084. DOI: 10.1021/jm100112j

[17] Haider MK. Computational analysis of protein-ligand interaction [disertation]. University of York: Department of Chemistry, 2010

[18] Böhm HJ, Schneider G. In: Mannhold R, Kubinyi H, Folkers G, editors. Protein-Ligand Interactions: From Molecular Recognition to Drug Design. Weinheim: Willey-VCH Verlag GmbH & Co KGaA; 2005. p. 234

[19] Mintseris J, Wiehe K, Pierce B, Anderson R, Chen R, Janin J, et al. Protein-protein docking benchmark 2.0: An update. Proteins: Structure, Function, and Bioinformatics. 2005;**60**(2):214-216. DOI: 10.1002/prot.20560

[20] Hwang H, Pierce B, Mintseris J, Janin J, Zhiping W. Protein-protein docking benchmark version 3.0. Proteins. 2008;**73**(3):169-172. DOI: 10.1002/prot.22106

[21] Tokunaga Y, Yamamori Y, Matubayasi N. Probabilistic analysis for identifying the driving force of protein folding. The Journal of Chemical Physics. 2018;(148):1-9. DOI: 10.1063/1.5019410

[22] Yan Z, Guo L, Hu L, Wang J. Specificity and affinity quantification of protein-protein interactions. Bioinformatics. 2013;**29**(9):1127-1133. DOI: 10.1093/bioinformatics/btt121

[23] Krüger DM, Garzón JI, Chacón P, Gohlke H. DrugScorePPI knowledge-based potentials used as scoring and objective function in protein-protein docking. PLoS ONE. 2014;**9**(2): 1-12. DOI: 10.1371/journal.pone.0089466

[24] Tobi D. Designing coarse grained- and atom based-potentials for protein-protein docking. BMC Structural Biology. 2010;**10**(40):1-11. DOI: 10.1186/1472-6807-10-40

[25] Chen F, Liu H, Sun H, Pan P, Li Y, Lia D, et al. Assessing the performance of the MM/PBSA and MM/GBSA methods. 6. Capability to predict protein-protein binding free energies and re-rank binding poses generated by protein-protein docking. Physical Chemistry Chemical Physics. 2016;**18**: 22129-22139. DOI: 10.1039/C6CP03670H

[26] Homeyer N, Gohlke H. Free energy calculations by the molecular mechanics Poisson-Boltzmann surface area method. Molecular Informatics. 2012;**31**(2):114-122. DOI: 10.1002/minf.201100135

[27] Chowdhury R, Rasheed M, Keidel D, Moussalem M, Olson A, Sanner M, et al. Protein-protein docking with F2Dock 2.0 and GB-Rerank. PLoS ONE. 2013;**8**(3):1-19. DOI: 10.1371/journal.pone.0051307

[28] Hou T, Wang J, Li Y, Wang W. Assessing the performance of the MM/PBSA and MM/GBSA methods. 1. The accuracy of binding free energy calculations based on Molecular dynamics simulations. Journal of

Chemical Information and Modeling. 2011:69-82. DOI: 10.1021/ci100275a

[29] Anishchenko I, Kundrotas PJ, Tuzikov AV, Vakser IA. Protein models docking benchmark 2. Proteins: Structure, Function and Bioinformatics. John Wiley Sons, Inc. 2015;**83**(5):891-897. DOI: 10.1002/prot.24784

[30] Takemura K, Guo K, Sakuraba H, Matubayasi S, Kitao N, Takemura A, Guo K, Sakuraba H, Matubayasi S, Nobuyuki. Evaluation of protein-protein docking model structures using all-atom molecular dynamics simulations combined with the solution theory in the energy representation. The Journal of Chemical Physics. 2012;**137**: v 215105-07 215101. DOI: 10.1063/1.4768901

[31] Raharjo SJ. In silico and In vitro analyses α- and γ-guaiene Pogostemon herbs for cyclooxygenase isoenzyme inhibitor. In Proceeding of International Conference of Essential Oil. 2017;**1**(1): 56-65

[32] Lovell SC, Davis IW, Arendall WB, Bakker PIW, Word JM, Prisant MG, Richardson JS, Richardson DC. Structure Validation by C α Geometry: φ/ψ and C β Deviation. Structure, Function, and Genetics. 2003;**50**(3): 437-450

[33] Campanera JM, Pouplana R. MMPBSA decomposition of the binding energy throughout a Molecular dynamics simulation of amyloid-Beta (Aß10−35) aggregation. Molecules. 2010;**15**:2730-2748. DOI: 10.3390/molecules15042730

[34] Sereda YV, Mansour AA and Ortoleva PJ. Virtual Molecular Dynamics. [thesis]. Indiana University, Bloomington: Department of Chemistry, I 2010

[35] Ossowska KK. Basic principles of Molecular dynamics (MD) theory. [thesis]. University of Strathclyde, 2012.

[36] Woo H, Roux B. Calculation of absolute protein—Ligand binding free. Proceedings of the National Academy of Sciences. 2005;**102**(19):6825-6830. DOI: 10.1073/pnas.040900510

[37] Uciechowska U, Schemies J, Neugebauer RC, Huda E-M, Schmitt ML, Meier R, et al. Thiobarbiturates as sirtuin inhibitors: Virtual screening, free-energy calculations, and biological testing. ChemMedChem. 2008;**94158**: 1965-1976. DOI: 10.1002/cmdc.200800104

[38] Haider MK, Bertrand H, Hubbard RE. Predicting fragment binding poses using a combined MCSS MM-GBSA approach. Journal of chemical information. 2010:A-N. DOI: 10.1021/ci100469n

[39] Raharjo SJ, Mahdi C, Nurdiana N, Kikuchi T, Fatchiyah F. In vitro and In silico: Selectivities of Seychellene compound as candidate cyclooxygenase isoenzyme inhibitor on pre-osteoblast cells. Current Enzyme Inhibition. 2017; **13**:2-10. DOI: 1875-6662/17

[40] Cer RZ, Mudunuri U, Stephens R, Lebeda FJ. IC_{50}-to-K_i: A web-based tool for converting IC_{50} to K_i values for inhibitors of enzyme activity and ligand binding. Nucleic Acids Research Advances. 2009;**1**(5):1-5. DOI: 10.1093/nar/gkp253

Chapter 5

Protein-Protein Docking Using Map Objects

Xiongwu Wu and Bernard R. Brooks

Abstract

Protein-protein docking is a molecular modeling strategy to predict biomolecular complexes and assemblies. Traditional protein-protein docking is performed at atomic resolution, which relies on X-ray and NMR experiments to provide structural information. When dealing with biomolecular assemblies of millions of atoms, atomic description of molecular objects becomes very computational inefficient. This article describes a development work that introduces map objects to molecular modeling studies to efficiently derive complex structures through map-map conformational search. This method has been implemented into CHARMM as the EMAP command and into AMBER in its SANDER program. This development enables molecular modeling and simulation to manipulate map objects, including map input, output, comparison, docking, etc. Through map objects, users can efficiently construct complex structures through protein-protein docking as well as from electron microscopy maps according to low map energies. Using a T-cell receptor (TCR) variable domain and acetylcholine binding protein (AChBP) as example systems, we showed the application to model an energetic optimized complex structure according to a complex map. The map objects serve as a bridge between high-resolution atomic structures and low-resolution image data.

Keywords: protein-protein docking, molecular modeling, electron microscopy, molecular image, computational tool, protein complexes, biomolecular assembly

1. Introduction

Protein-protein docking has been a powerful approach to provide structural insights into biological procedures at atomic level [1–4]. Based on the structural information provided by X-ray and NMR, as well as constraints derived from biological data such as mutagenesis observations, protein-protein docking can produce structures and interactions of protein complexes, which helps to illustrate structural mechanism of many biological processes [5–7].

New development in experimental technologies, such as electron microscopy, provides an approach to obtain low-resolution structure information of large molecules and their assemblies [8]. Extracting structure information from these low-resolution maps and obtaining atomic interpretation of the large biomolecular assemblies become a central piece of modern structural biology [9]. This requires molecular modeling to be conducted on these low-resolution maps, as well as high-resolution atomic structures, to maximize the capability in structural biology studies.

On the other hand, as the development of structural biology, molecular modeling is applied to larger and larger biomolecular machineries. As the biology systems become larger, atomic description of molecular system becomes very inefficient and time-consuming. Millions of atoms and their chemical structural become redundant in many of modeling studies. Therefore, it would be very efficient if large biomolecules are simplified to shape objects while ignoring their internal structures. Although molecular flexibility plays important roles in biological activities, in many cases, molecular geometric shapes plus surface properties are sufficient to describe many cellular processes such as molecule assembling and protein-protein binding. In these cases, it is satisfactory to describe large molecules as rigid domains. In some cases certain internal flexibility can be simplified to the motion of several rigid fragments. Therefore, molecular modeling of large biomolecular machinery can be achieved efficiently by simplifying biomolecules with simplified shape objects.

In this work, we introduce map objects to represent molecules with fixed structures to achieve efficient molecular modeling of large molecular systems and to efficiently derive structural information from low-resolution experimental maps. Map objects are designed to work with high-resolution atomic structures so that low-resolution maps are interchangeable with high-resolution atomic structures. A map object represents a property distribution over certain space, while a molecular structure is generally described by the coordinates of a set of atoms. This work describes an efficient approach to handle and manipulate map objects so that efficient molecular modeling of large systems can be performed.

2. Method and design

We introduce map objects to represent space occupation of molecular structures. Unlike chemical description of molecules that contain atoms that are linked by

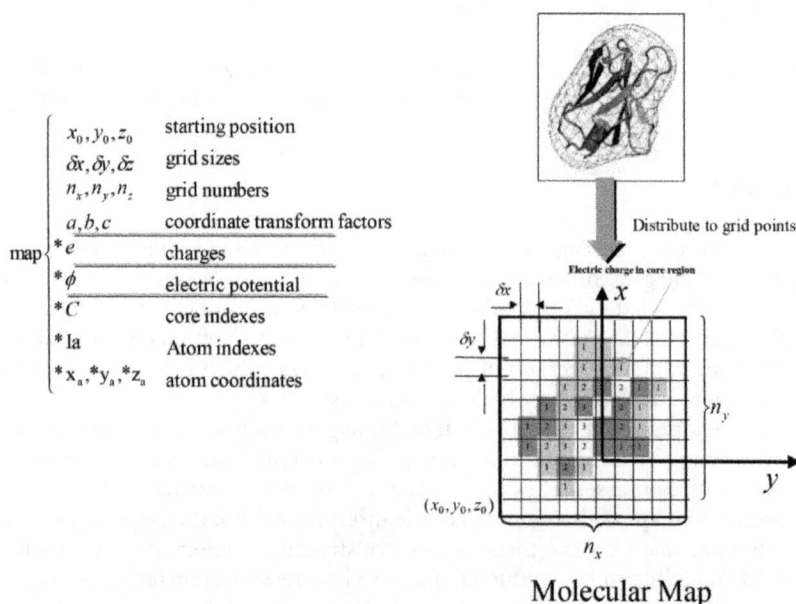

Figure 1.
A map object and its properties.

chemical bonds, a map does not have internal chemical structures. Instead, a map represents a spatial distribution of certain properties, typically electron density. This distribution generally is described as scalar values at discrete grid points due to irregularity of the distributions and limit in storage. **Figure 1** shows a cartoon of a map object. As can be seen, a map objects contains three components.

2.1 Grid definition

The grid of a map object is defined by its starting position, $x0$, $y0$, and $z0$; grid intervals, dx, dy, and dz; and grid point numbers, nx, ny, and nz.

2.2 Molecular reference

Because we use map to represent a molecular structure, we use molecular reference to record which molecule this map is representing. Through reference molecule, map object and molecule coordinates become interchangeable.

2.3 Distribution properties

The distribution property describes the distribution of given property over the space covered by the grid points. This can be the electron density measured in experiment or properties generated from reference molecules.

Here are several typical types of map objects used in molecular modeling:

1. Electron density maps

This is the most widely used map type, which describes the electron density over the space. This type of map is often determined from electron microscopy. It can also be derived from molecular structure based on atomic coordinates and type.

2. Electric charge maps

This type of map is solely derived from molecular structures based on a force field. The partial charges of atoms are distributed to their nearest grid points.

3. Electric field maps

Because electrostatic interactions are long ranged, it is difficult to have a map to cover a very large space. Instead, we propose to use transformed coordinates:

$$X = \frac{x}{|x| + b}, \tag{1}$$

$$x = \frac{bX}{1 - |X|}, \tag{2}$$

where x is the real space coordinate, X is the reduced coordinate, and b is a constant controlling the reduction. X will take a range of $(-1, 1)$ to represent a real space of x over $(-\infty, \infty)$.

4. VDW core maps

The VDW cores provide boundary to avoid overlapping between molecules. The core map is constructed based on the accessibility of a molecular structure. The surface has low core index, while the center has high index (the core indices are shown as the number in each grid box in **Figure 1**).

2.4 Rigid domains

Because a map object contains a large amount of data, it is inconvenient to perform movement on a map itself. For example, a rotation of a map object will result in the rectangular space not parallel to the coordinate axis anymore, and new boundaries and distributions need be updated accordingly. In addition, a real system often contains more than one copy of some molecular species, and it would be very memory costing to have a map object for each copy of these species. Instead, we define a rigid domain to represent a copy of the molecular species. A rigid domain contains only the identity of the map object it represents and the position and orientation vectors related to the map object, and can be manipulated easily. A rigid domain can be understood as a mobile representation of a map object. Each rigid domain has a unique identity, and many rigid domains can represent the same map object. **Figure 2** shows the map objects of the α-chain and β-chain of a TCR variable domain and their manipulation through rigid domains.

Each rigid domain is defined by its map ID and its translation vector, **T**, and rotational matrix, **U**:

$$\mathbf{T} = \begin{pmatrix} t_x \\ t_y \\ t_z \end{pmatrix}, \mathbf{U} = \begin{pmatrix} u_{11} & u_{12} & u_{13} \\ u_{21} & u_{22} & u_{23} \\ u_{31} & u_{32} & u_{33} \end{pmatrix} \tag{3}$$

The operation, translation, and rotation are done by applying these vectors:

$$\mathbf{T}^{(i+1)} = \mathbf{T}^{(i)} + \Delta\mathbf{T}^{(i+1)} = \begin{pmatrix} t_x^{(i)} \\ t_y^{(i)} \\ t_z^{(i)} \end{pmatrix} + \begin{pmatrix} \Delta t_x^{(i+1)} \\ \Delta t_y^{(i+1)} \\ \Delta t_z^{(i+1)} \end{pmatrix} \tag{4}$$

$$\mathbf{U}^{(i+1)} = \Omega^{(i+1)} \times \mathbf{U}^{(i)} = \begin{pmatrix} \omega_{11}^{(i+1)} & \omega_{11}^{(i+1)} & \omega_{13}^{(i+1)} \\ \omega_{21}^{(i+1)} & \omega_{22}^{(i+1)} & \omega_{23}^{(i+1)} \\ \omega_{31}^{(i+1)} & \omega_{32}^{(i+1)} & \omega_{33}^{(i+1)} \end{pmatrix} \times \begin{pmatrix} u_{11}^{(i)} & u_{11}^{(i)} & u_{13}^{(i)} \\ u_{21}^{(i)} & u_{22}^{(i)} & u_{23}^{(i)} \\ u_{31}^{(i)} & u_{32}^{(i)} & u_{33}^{(i)} \end{pmatrix} \tag{5}$$

and many operations can be accumulated without losing accuracy:

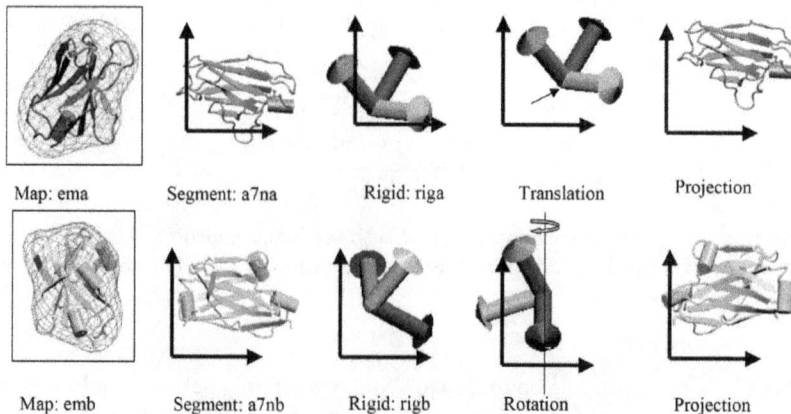

| Map: ema | Segment: a7na | Rigid: riga | Translation | Projection |
| Map: emb | Segment: a7nb | Rigid: rigb | Rotation | Projection |

Figure 2.
Rigid domains as a convenient way to manipulate map objects.

$$T^{(n)} = T^{(n-1)} + \Delta T^{(n)} = T^{(n-2)} + \Delta T^{(n)} + \Delta T^{(n-1)} = T^0) + \sum_{i=1}^{n} \Delta T^{(i)} \qquad (6)$$

$$U^{(n)} = \Omega^{(n)} \times U^{(n-1)} = \Omega^{(n)} \times \Omega^{(n-1)} \times U^{(n-2)} = \prod_{i=1}^{n} \Omega^{(i)} \times U^{(0)} \qquad (7)$$

When a map object is created, a rigid domain at origin is created for it, with

$$T = \begin{pmatrix} 0 \\ 0 \\ 0 \end{pmatrix}, U = \begin{pmatrix} 1 & 0 & 0 \\ 0 & 1 & 0 \\ 0 & 0 & 1 \end{pmatrix} \qquad (8)$$

A rigid domain can also be created for a molecular structure by linking the structure to a given map object according to the translation vector and rotation matrix from the reference coordinates to the linked structure.

$$X = T + U \times X^{(ref)} \qquad (9)$$

This equation also provides a way to update the structure coordinates according to the position and orientation of a rigid domain.

2.5 Map comparison

Map comparison provides a target function for fitting one map into another map. Four types of cross-correlation functions [10] are provided for comparison between map objects, which are listed below.

1. Density correlation (DC)

$$DC_{mn} = \frac{\overline{\rho_m \rho_n} - \overline{\rho_m}\,\overline{\rho_n}}{\delta(\rho_m)\delta(\rho_n)} \qquad (10)$$

where

$$\overline{\rho} = \frac{1}{n_x n_y n_z} \sum_{i}^{n_x} \sum_{j}^{n_y} \sum_{k}^{n_z} \rho(i,j,k) \qquad (11)$$

and

$$\delta(\rho) = \sqrt{\overline{\rho^2} - \overline{\rho}^2} \qquad (12)$$

represent the average and fluctuation of the density distribution. DC_{mn} is the density correlation of map m to map n. **Figure 3** shows two comparison maps in two dimensions. DC_{mn} is calculated according to map m's dimension and grid properties. The calculation runs over all grid points of map m, which are transformed and interpolated into grid points of map n to get corresponding density properties.

2. Laplacian correlation (LC)

$$LC_{mn} = \frac{\overline{\nabla^2 \rho_m \nabla^2 \rho_n} - \overline{\nabla^2 \rho_m}\,\overline{\nabla^2 \rho_n}}{\delta(\nabla^2 \rho_m)\delta(\nabla^2 \rho_n)} \qquad (13)$$

where $\nabla^2 \rho$ is the Laplacian filtered density derived from density distribution by the following finite difference approximation:

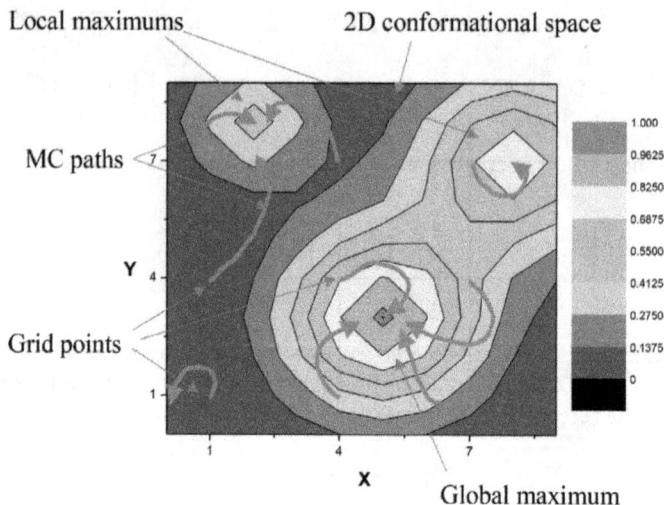

Figure 3.
A cartoon to show the grid-threading Monte Carlo searching method.

$$\nabla^2 \rho_{ijk} = \rho_{i+1jk} + \rho_{i-1jk} + \rho_{ij+1k} + \rho_{ij-1k} + \rho_{ijk+1} + \rho_{ijk-1} - 6\rho_{ijk} \tag{14}$$

LC_{mn} is the Laplacian correlation of map m to map n. Similar to DC_{mn}, LC_{mn} is calculated according to map m's dimension and grid properties.

3. Core-weighted density correlation (CWDC)

$$CWDC_{mn} = \frac{\overline{(\rho_m \rho_n)}_w - \overline{(\rho_m)}_w \overline{(\rho_n)}_w}{\delta_w(\rho_m)\delta_w(\rho_n)} \tag{15}$$

where $\overline{(X)}_w$ represents a core-weighted average of distribution property X:

$$\overline{(X)}_w = \frac{\sum_{i,j,k} w_{mn}(i,j,k) X(i,j,k)}{\sum_{i,j,k} w_{mn}(i,j,k)} \tag{16}$$

and

$$\delta_w(X) = \sqrt{\overline{(X^2)}_w - \overline{(X)}_w^2}, \tag{17}$$

$$w_{mn} = \frac{f_m^a}{f_m^a + k_c f_n^a + b} \tag{18}$$

where w_{mm} is core-weighting function of core m to core n. Three parameters, a, b, and kc, control the dependence of the function to the core indices. We chose $a = 2$ and $kc = 1$ in this work calculations, and b is set to a very small value, say 10–6, to ensure $w_{mn} = 0$ when $f_m = 0$ and $f_n = 0$. Therefore, only the core region of map m has contribution to the core-weighted density correlation, $CWDC_{mn}$.

4. Core-weighted Laplacian correlation (CWLC)

$$CWLC_{mn} = \frac{\overline{(\nabla^2 \rho_m \nabla^2 \rho_n)}_w - \overline{(\nabla^2 \rho_m)}_w \overline{(\nabla^2 \rho_n)}_w}{\delta_w(\nabla^2 \rho_m)\delta_w(\nabla^2 \rho_n)} \tag{19}$$

$CWLC_{mn}$ uses Laplacian filtered density, instead of the density in the calculation. Again, only the core region of map m has contribution to the core-weighted Laplacian correlation, $CWLC_{mn}$.

2.6 Molecular interactions between map objects

Energetics of molecular systems is the basis of molecular modeling. Calculation of molecular interaction using map objects is the crucial step for a successful modeling or simulation study. For atomic objects interaction calculation is pairwise and is very time-consuming for large molecular assemblies. For map objects, we propose to use field interactions that can be calculated much more efficiently. We define four types of interactions to describe interaction between map objects: electric field interaction, surface charge-charge interaction, VDW interaction, and desolvation interaction as described below.

1. Electric field interaction

The electric field around a molecule is described by the field map with scaled coordinates. The interaction with the field is

$$\overset{ele}{\underset{12}{E}} = \sum_{m_1} e_1 \varphi_1 \tag{20}$$

where e_1 is the charge at the charge map 1 and φ_2 is the electric field from object 2, which depends on the dielectric constant, ε, and distances from each grid points of object 2. The dielectric constant, $\varepsilon = 80$, is used for most cases.

2. VDW interaction

Surface interaction brings the surface together while avoiding core overlapping. The surface can be identified by low core index. We propose to use the following equation to make the surface contact favorable while overlapping unfavorable:

$$\overset{vdw}{\underset{12}{E}} = 4v \frac{\delta_1^2}{\delta_2^2} \sum_{m_1} \left(\left(\frac{C_1 C_2}{3} \right)^2 - \frac{C_1 C_2}{3} \right) \tag{21}$$

where C1 and C2 are the core indices of molecular 1 and 2 at each grid point and δ_1 and δ_2 are the grid intervals of map. 1 and 2, respectively. v is the VDW interaction parameter.

3. Surface charge: charge interaction

Upon binding, the surface charge groups will contact with each other. The surface charge–charge interaction is different from the charge-field interaction which is screened by the solvent environment:

$$\overset{binding}{\underset{12}{E}} = b \frac{\delta_1^2}{\sqrt{\delta_1^3 \delta_2^3}} \sum_{m_1} e_1 e_2 \tag{22}$$

where b is the surface interaction parameter.

4. Desolvation interaction

Before and after binding, the surface charge groups change from the solvation state to the buried state and will create an energy gain we termed as desolvation energy:

$$E_{12}^{desolv} = s\delta_1^2 \sum_{m_1} \left(\frac{C_1 e_1^2}{\delta_1^3 \left(1 + (C_1/2)^6\right)\left(1 + C_2^6\right)} - \frac{C_2 e_2^2}{\delta_2^3 \left(1 + C_1^6\right)\left(1 + (C_2/2)^6\right)} \right) \quad (23)$$

where s is the desolvation parameter.

These interaction parameters used to define the interactions, Eqs. (20)–(23), can be derived from atomic force field or from experimental data. By fitting into energies calculated with the CHARMM force field [11], we obtained the parameters $v = 0.14$ kcalÅ, $b = 330$ kcal/(C^{2}Å), and $s = 70$ kcal/(C^{2}Å^2).

2.7 Conformational search

We implemented the grid-threading Monte Carlo searching algorithm [10] for robustly fitting rigid domains to a target map. The grid-threading Monte Carlo (GTMC) search is a combination of the grid search and Monte Carlo sampling. As shown in **Figure 3**, the conformational space is split into grid points, and short Monte Carlo searches are performed to identify local maximums around the grid points. The global maximum is identified among the local minimums.

3. Results and discussions

3.1 Complex structures from EM maps

Deriving high-resolution molecular assembly structures from microscopy maps are a major application of the map approach. This method has been successfully applied into several experimental studies [12, 13]. **Figure 4** illustrates the steps to perform a fitting of high-resolution molecular structure into electron

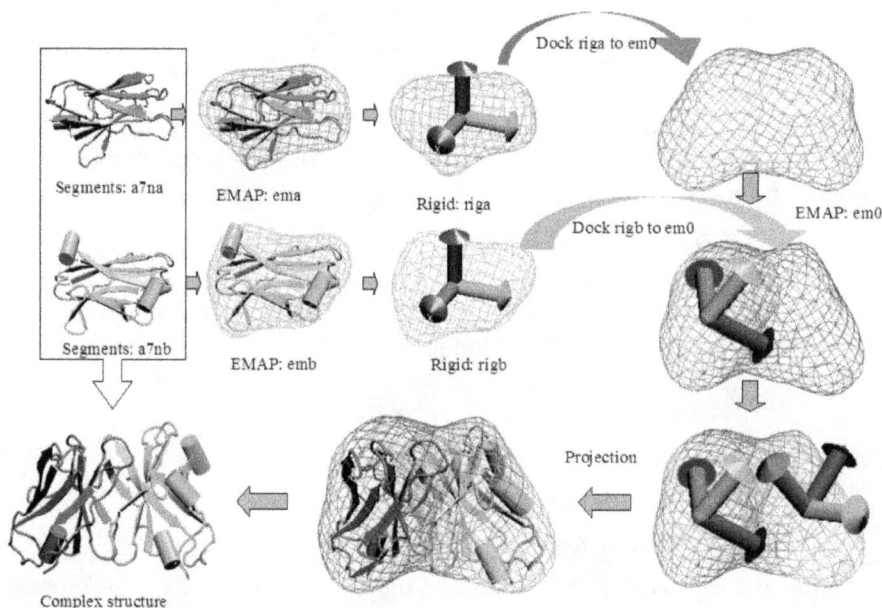

Figure 4.
Steps to derive molecular assembly structures by fitting molecular structures into electron microscopy maps.

microscopy maps. We chose a T-cell receptor (TCR) variable domain (PDB code: 1a7n) as an example complex to illustrate the modeling process with map objects. The TCR variable domain is a complex of two chains, α-chain and β-chain. The two chains are first blurred into maps of the same resolution (here 15 Å) as the EM map. Then each map is fitted into the EM map to get a complex map. The complex map is projected back to atomic structures, which is the complex structure we are looking for. The root mean square (rms) deviation of the fitting result from X-ray complex is 3 Å.

The structure obtained from map fitting generally is not optimized in atomic details. There are often atom overlaps or improper spacing between components. This structural mismatch can be removed by many modeling methods available in CHARMM [14, 15], such as energy minimization and simulated annealing, if the fitting result is very close to the right structure. After the minimization, the rms deviation is 0.97 Å.

3.2 Complex structures from energy optimization

The energy function is designed to have the minimum at the binding conformation. Therefore, it is possible to determine complex structures through minimizing the map interaction energy in cases where the EM complex map is not available. It should be noted that the map object assumes certain rigidity of a molecular object. Certain flexibility of loop region can be accommodated by the low-resolution characters, while large flexibilities like domain movement should be dealt with multiple map objects. Recently, this method was successfully applied in modeling of the peroxiredoxin (Prx) complex [16].

Figure 5 shows the steps to perform an energy-based conformational search to determine complex structures. In this case, no EM map is used. The TCR chains are transferred into property maps that allow interaction between map objects to be

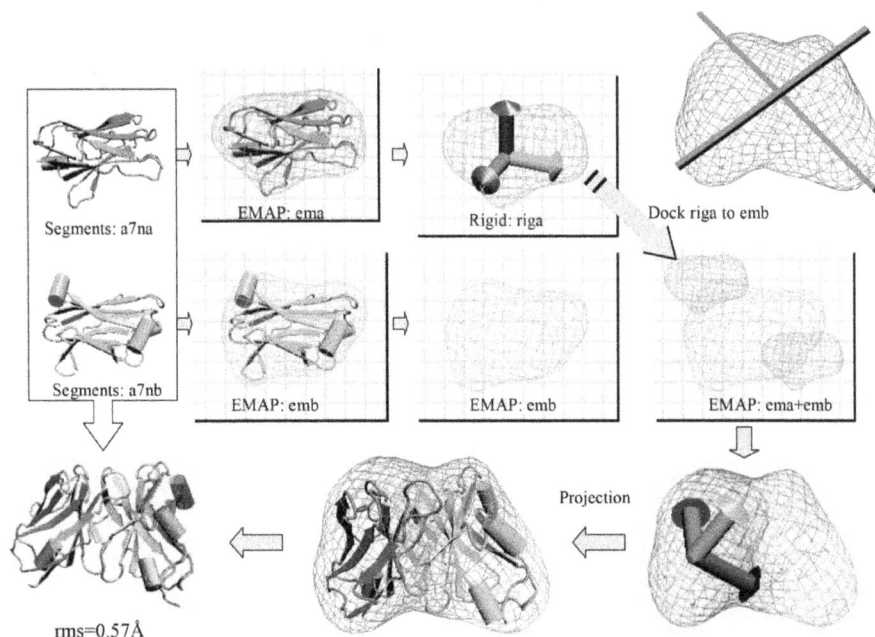

Figure 5.
Derive complex structure base on map interactions.

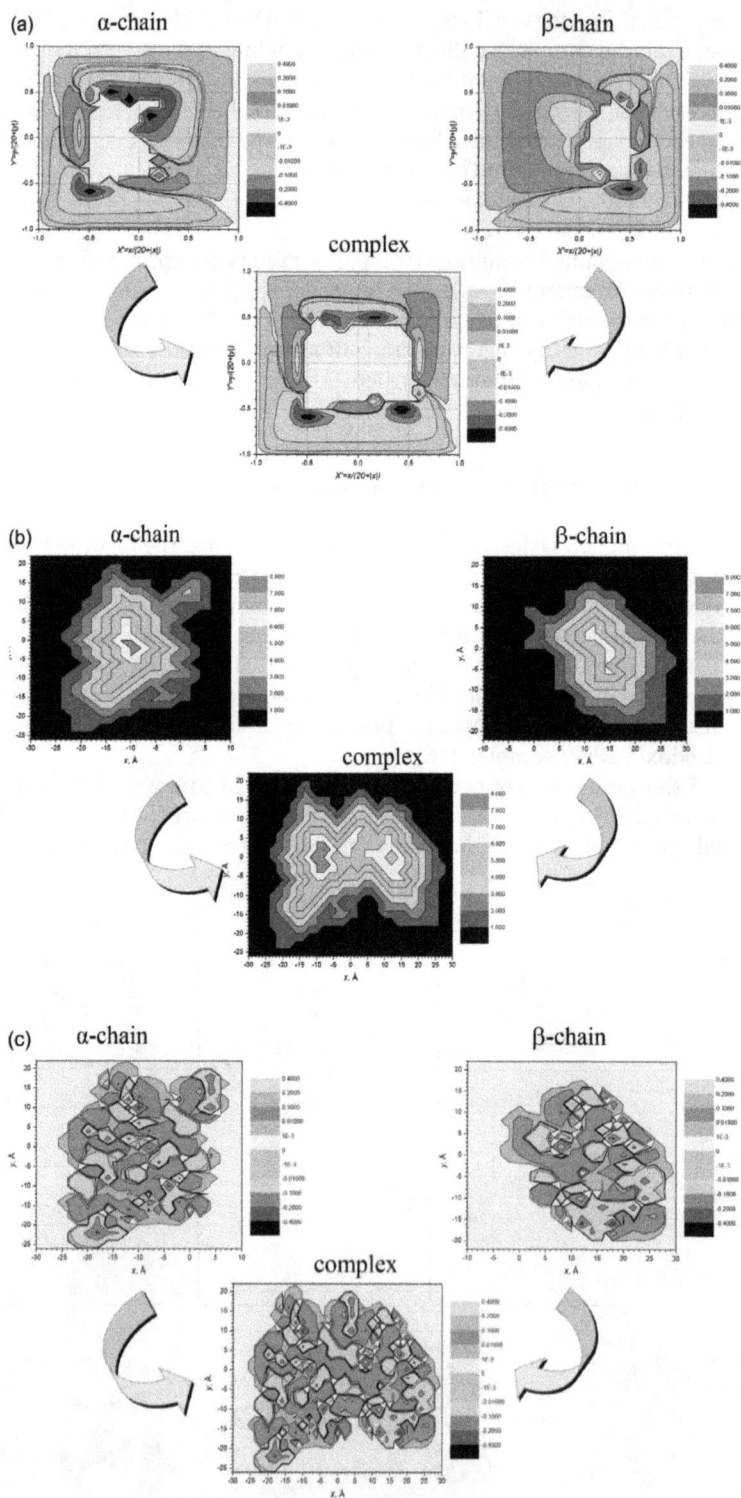

Figure 6.
(a) Electrostatic field maps of TCR two chains and complexes. (b) Core-index maps of TCR two chains and complex. (c) Partial charge maps of TCR two chains and complexes.

calculated. By searching the minimum interaction energy conformation, the complex structure is determined. The final result is only 0.57 Å away from the X-ray structure. It should be noted that this is an ideal case that the structure of the two chains is taken from the complex and there is no conformational change in this fitting process.

It is interesting to see that energy-based approach to derive complex structure takes account of molecular structure and energetic information of molecules. **Figure 6a–c** shows the electric field, shape, and charge maps of the two chains and their complex. Obviously, the two chains are binding together to have the low potential region matching the high potential one, to have shape complementary to each other, and to have surface charge overlapped oppositely.

Figure 6a shows the electric field of TCR α-chain and β-chain and their complex. Please notice the reduced coordinates are used for the map. The range of $(-1, 1)$ for the reduced coordinates covers the range of $(-\infty, \infty)$ for the regular coordinates. The α-chain has negative field near its top-left and bottom-right areas and positive field near its lower-right and upper-left areas. Correspondingly, the β-chain has positive field at its top-right area and negative field at its bottom area, which are complementary to the α-chain. As a result, the complex map has negative field at its top and bottom areas and positive field at its left and right areas. The symmetric distribution of the field of the complex indicates its stability.

Figure 6b shows the core indices of TCR α-chain and β-chain and their complex. The high values in the core indices indicate the region further away from surface and are difficult to access. The α-chain and β-chain that show complementary shape are the binding surface. Their complexes are the two maps matching together.

Figure 6c shows the electric charge distribution of TCR α-chain and β-chain and their complex. The α-chain map shows more negative charges at the right side, while the β-chain shows more positive charges at its left side. The complex map shows the two chains come together with negative patches contacting positive patches. Overall, these map interactions provide energetic basis for protein-protein docking as shown in **Figure 5**.

As a further example of protein-protein docking, we show the procedure to build the pentamer of acetylcholine binding protein (AChBP). The monomers

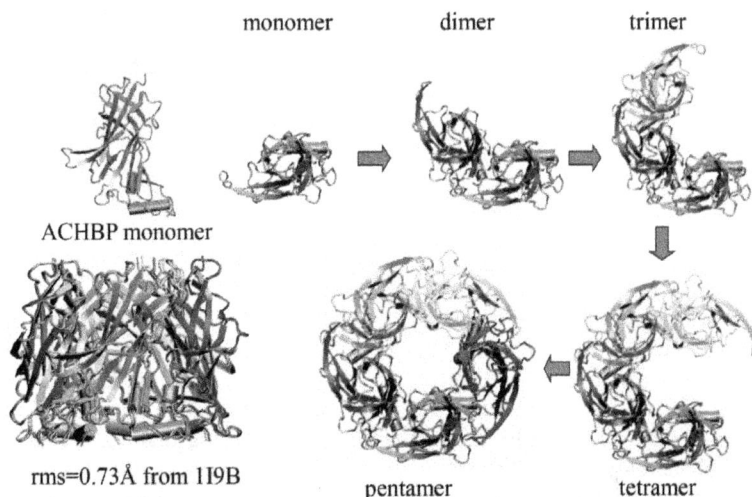

Figure 7.
Protein-protein docking of acetylcholine binding protein (AChBP) to build its pentamer.

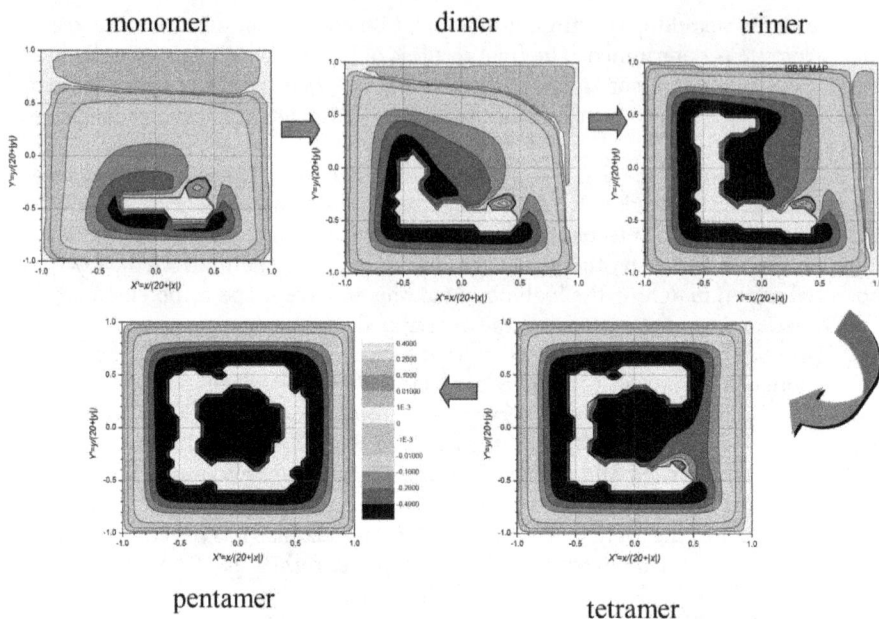

Figure 8.
Electric field map at each docking stage to build the pentamer of acetylcholine binding protein (AChBP).

are docked one by one to form dimer, trimer, tetramer, and pentamer (**Figure 7**). The resulting pentamer is only 0.73 Å away from the X-ray structure, 1I9B. The electric field maps during the building process are shown in **Figure 8**. From the field map of the monomer, we can see the most positive field is at the top-right area and the most negative field is at the bottom-left area. A dimer is formed by matching the positive area of the second monomer with the negative area of the first one. The third monomer's positive area fits into the most negative area of the dimer to form the trimer. Similarly, the fourth and fifth monomers are docked to form the tetramer and pentamer. The map interaction limits the way of docking monomers and allows correct assemblies to be built.

Map objects cannot only be used to model rigid proteins [17], they can also be used for targeted conformational search such as flexible fitting and restrained molecular dynamics [18, 19]. Map objects provide an efficient bridge from molecular systems to large-scale bodies such as cells and organelles.

4. Conclusions

This work designed and developed a computational tool to manipulate map information for molecular modeling studies. Protein–protein docking can be efficiently performed with map objects. This tool is implemented into CHARMM, as a module, EMAP, and into AMBER in its SANDER program. Our design and implementation make it very flexible and efficient to perform various manipulations of map objects and to perform some routine task related to map data. This module enables user to construct macromolecular assemblies by docking high-resolution X-ray or NMR structures to low-resolution cryo-electron microscopy maps. And when there is no EM map available, this module allows user to search for low-energy complex structures, for example, in protein-protein docking. By replacing high-resolution atomic structure with low-resolution map objects, this work creates a convenient approach to extend the molecular modeling studies to large biomolecular machinery. This map-based approach can extend modeling and simulation objects from molecular systems to macroscopic systems like cells and bacteria.

Acknowledgements

This research was supported by the Intramural Research Programs of National Heart, Lung, and Blood Institute (Z01 HL001027-34).

Conflict of interest

The authors declare there is no conflict of interest in publishing this work.

Author details

Xiongwu Wu* and Bernard R. Brooks
Laboratory of Computational Biology, NHLBI, NIH, Bethesda, MD, USA

*Address all correspondence to: wuxw@nhlbi.nih.gov

IntechOpen

References

[1] Nadaradjane AA, Guerois R, Andreani J. Protein-protein docking using evolutionary information. Methods in Molecular Biology. 2018; **1764**:429-447

[2] Moal IH, Chaleil RAG, Bates PA. Flexible protein-protein docking with SwarmDock. Methods in Molecular Biology. 2018;**1764**:413-428

[3] Kaczor AA, Bartuzi D, Stepniewski TM, Matosiuk D, Selent J. Protein-protein docking in drug design and discovery. Methods in Molecular Biology. 2018;**1762**:285-305

[4] Zhang Q, Feng T, Xu L, Sun H, Pan P, Li Y, et al. Recent advances in protein-protein docking. Current Drug Targets. 2016;**17**(14):1586-1594

[5] Matsuzaki Y, Ohue M, Uchikoga N, Akiyama Y. Protein-protein interaction network prediction by using rigid-body docking tools: Application to bacterial chemotaxis. Protein and Peptide Letters. 2014;**21**(8):790-798

[6] Gaur M, Tiwari A, Chauhan RP, Pandey D, Kumar A. Molecular modeling, docking and protein-protein interaction analysis of MAPK signalling cascade involved in Camalexin biosynthesis in *Brassica rapa*. Bioinformation. 2018;**14**(4):145-152

[7] Meyerson JR, Kumar J, Chittori S, Rao P, Pierson J, Bartesaghi A, et al. Structural mechanism of glutamate receptor activation and desensitization. Nature. 2014;**514**(7522):328-334

[8] Subramaniam S, Bartesaghi A, Liu J, Bennett AE, Sougrat R. Electron tomography of viruses. Current Opinion in Structural Biology. 2007;**17**(5): 596-602

[9] Bartesaghi A, Subramaniam S. Membrane protein structure determination using cryo-electron tomography and 3D image averaging. Current Opinion in Structural Biology. 2009;**19**(4):402-407

[10] Wu X, Milne JL, Borgnia MJ, Rostapshov AV, Subramaniam S, Brooks BR. A core-weighted fitting method for docking atomic structures into low-resolution maps: Application to cryo-electron microscopy. Journal of Structural Biology. 2003;**141**(1):63-76

[11] MacKerell AD, Bashford D, Bellott M, Dunbrack RL, Evanseck JD, Field MJ, et al. All-atom empirical potential for molecular modeling and dynamics studies of proteins. The Journal of Physical Chemistry. B. 1998;**102**(18): 3586-3616

[12] Milne JL, Wu X, Borgnia MJ, Lengyel JS, Brooks BR, Shi D, et al. Molecular structure of a 9-MDa icosahedral pyruvate dehydrogenase subcomplex containing the E2 and E3 enzymes using cryoelectron microscopy. The Journal of Biological Chemistry. 2006;**281**(7):4364-4370

[13] Milne JL, Shi D, Rosenthal PB, Sunshine JS, Domingo GJ, Wu X, et al. Molecular architecture and mechanism of an icosahedral pyruvate dehydrogenase complex: A multifunctional catalytic machine. The EMBO Journal. 2002;**21**(21):5587-5598

[14] Brooks BR, Brooks CL 3rd, Mackerell AD Jr, Nilsson L, Petrella RJ, Roux B, et al. CHARMM: The biomolecular simulation program. Journal of Computational Chemistry. 2009;**30**(10):1545-1614

[15] Brooks BR, Bruccoleri RE, Olafson BD, States DJ, Swaminathan S, Jaun B, et al. CHARMM: A program for macromolecular energy, minimization, and dynamics calculations. Journal of

Computational Chemistry. 1983;**4**: 187-217

[16] Lee DY, Park SJ, Jeong W, Sung HJ, Oho T, Wu X, et al. Mutagenesis and modeling of the peroxiredoxin (Prx) complex with the NMR structure of ATP-bound human sulfiredoxin implicate aspartate 187 of Prx I as the catalytic residue in ATP hydrolysis. Biochemistry. 2006;**45**(51):15301-15309

[17] Wright JD, Sargsyan K, Wu X, Brooks BR, Lim C. Protein–protein docking using EMAP in CHARMM and support vector machine: Application to Ab/Ag complexes. Journal of Chemical Theory and Computation. 2013;**9**(9): 4186-4194

[18] Wu X, Subramaniam S, Case DA, Wu KW, Brooks BR. Targeted conformational search with map-restrained self-guided Langevin dynamics: Application to flexible fitting into electron microscopic density maps. Journal of Structural Biology. 2013; **183**(3):429-440

[19] Bartesaghi A, Aguerrebere C, Falconieri V, Banerjee S, Earl LA, Zhu X, et al. Atomic resolution cryo-EM structure of β-galactosidase. Structure. 2018;**26**(6):848-856

Chapter 6

Computational Study of Radiopharmaceuticals

Emine Selin Demir, Emre Ozgenc, Meliha Ekinci,
Evren Atlihan Gundogdu, Derya İlem Özdemir
and Makbule Asikoglu

Abstract

Radiopharmaceuticals contain radionuclides and pharmaceuticals. Research on radiopharmaceuticals has been increasing in recent years by increasing the importance of early diagnosis in diseases. It is generally accepted that investigation and development of new radiopharmaceuticals are time and resource consuming. Computational methods have provided exciting contributions to pharmaceutical research and development. The need for designing new radiopharmaceutical drugs enhances the importance of computational programs. At this point, the structure, chemical, physical and physicochemical properties of molecules should be predicted/evaluated by using computational methods. While these methods obtain useful estimates, they make it easier for researchers and clinicians to make the right choices. Also, by providing accurate and effective results, they contribute to reduce the cost of research and can be used to simulate complex biochemical situations before research helping us to avoid harmful effects of drugs. In this study, authors emphasis about radiopharmaceuticals and the computational tools related to the development of new radiopharmaceuticals.

Keywords: computational method, radiopharmaceutical

1. Radiopharmaceuticals

Radiopharmaceuticals are radioactive drugs that can be used either for diagnostic or therapeutic purposes in nuclear medicine applications. In nuclear medicine, 95% of radiopharmaceuticals are used in diagnosis and 5% of them in therapeutic usage [1, 2]. The pharmaceutical component directs radioactivity to the target site of the body (disease regions, organs). A radionuclide emits detectable signals from outside the organism for visualization or delivers therapeutic levels of radiation dose to target sites. Radiopharmaceuticals are bound to accumulate in certain organs or tissues according to the physical, chemical and biological properties of the pharmaceutical part [1]. They are not chemically distinguishable from non-radioactive analogues and participate in biochemical events in the organism [2]. Organ functions can be visualized by the radiation emitted by radionuclides in their structure. A pathological change that can lead/leading to abnormal function can be diagnosed at the molecular level without going to the morphological level. So, diseases can be treated quickly after imaging [1].

With the widespread use of radiopharmaceuticals, the need for specialized pharmacists as known radiopharmacists has increased. Radiopharmaceuticals should be prepared by radiopharmacists and administered by clinicians to the patient. The doses of radiopharmaceuticals are defined either millicurie or microcurie. The pharmaceutical form of the radiopharmaceuticals may be solutions, kit, capsules and aerosols. The amount of active substance in the radiopharmaceutical is at a low dose that does not have a pharmacological effect. The shelf life of a radiopharmaceutical depends on half-life of radionuclide. Quality control of radiopharmaceuticals should be done before administration to patients.

A radiopharmaceutical optimal performance should have some characteristics. While the radiopharmaceuticals used for diagnosis emit gamma ray, the radiopharmaceuticals used for treatment emit beta ray. Alpha and beta radiation, which have particle radiation, are not desirable for diagnosis due to high linear energy transfers (LET). Because this energy is completely absorbed in the body, some particles that can escape to the body and cannot reach the crystal in the imaging system [3].

The ideal radionuclide energy for imaging should be around 100–300 kilo electron volts (keV). The quality of image falls when it is above or below these energy values. In radiopharmaceuticals used for treatment, the energy should be higher than above 1 MeV.

Ideally, the effective half-life of a radiopharmaceutical should be greater than about 1.5 times the imaging time. This pro vides a good image between the maximum dose and the minimum dose that can be injected into the patient, so that the counting statistics and image quality are optimal. On the other hand, the effective half-life of radiopharmaceuticals used in treatment is indicated by hours and days.

The localization of radiopharmaceuticals should be high in the desired organs or tissues. Low dose for both, patient and personnel, is necessary of ideal radiopharmaceutical. When the radioactivity ratio in the target/non-target area is low and the radiation dose increases in non-target areas, treatment or diagnosis efficiency of radiopharmaceuticals decreases. They must be non-toxic, sterile and pyrogen-free for patient compliance. Finally, radiopharmaceuticals must maintain their chemical stability during usage, should be cheap and easy to find, easy to prepare and appropriate quality controls [4].

2. Classification of radiopharmaceuticals

In general, four types of radiopharmaceuticals are used in medical practice. The first of these is ready to use radiopharmaceuticals. These products have a shelf life. Administration to the patient is performed after the radioactive decay is calculated. Iodine (I-123) capsules, I-131 hippurane, Gallium (Ga-67) citrate, Tallium (Tl-201) chloride, Xsenone (Xe-133) aerosol, Technetium (Tc-99 m) pertechnetate are the examples of this group. The second type of radiopharmaceuticals is radiopharmaceuticals obtained from semi-manufactured products. They are prepared by combining the kits with radionuclides that obtained from the generator. The third type of radiopharmaceuticals is prepared directly before use. Products of this group should be prepared and used immediately. Examples of this group are the particle accelerator products. The fourth type of radiopharmaceuticals is based on preparation of samples taken from the patient. The patient's cell or plasma proteins are radiolabeled with radionuclide and given to the same patient. An example of this group is Tc-99 m radiolabelled WBC. The laboratories have different regulations and rules because of this, radiolabelling efficiency and cell viability should be checked for this group after radiolabeling process [5].

3. Computational models for drug development

Every patient and disease are different. The personalized treatment approach can be better for each patient requires. The development of individual mechanistic models of the disease process offers the possibility of attaining truly personalized drug-based therapy and diagnosis. At this point, computational methods have provided exciting contributions to pharmaceutical research and development. The need for individual drug design enhances the importance of computational models. Infrared (IR), ultraviolet (UV) and nuclear magnetic resonance (NMR) spectra of the molecule to be predicted, are important and generated by computational approaches in order to characterize molecular structure. The compatibility of the target protein active site with the small molecule (or ligand) is examined, so more effective molecules could be designed by this way [6].

Computer-aided drug design has been established as a valuable tool for the design of new molecules, with many success stories since the 1980s. Pharmaceutical companies have invested substantially in bioinformatics approaches, and it has been predicted that such methodologies will have an important role in pharmacogenomics and personalized medicine. The American Food and Drug Administration (FDA) accepted and expressed the importance of new biomarkers and radiopharmaceuticals for personalizing treatments [7].

Mathematical models of drug design are used to guide drug research and development. Computational models provide the identification of the factors involved in the absorption, distribution, metabolism, elimination and access to the target region of the chemical components. It also exposes the dynamics involved in the interaction of the compounds with the target (receptor, enzyme, etc.,). These models are effective in analyzing the fate of drugs that have undergone biotransformation. It helps us to comment on the undesirable effects or toxic effects of drugs and to help us explain drug-drug interactions. The concept of virtual clinical trials and the integrated use of *in silico*, *in vitro* and *in vivo* models in preclinical development could lead to significant gains in efficiency and order of magnitude increases in the cost effectiveness of drug development and approval [8].

The targeting agent is used as a starting point for the design of computer-assisted drug active substance. Examples of targeting agents include receptors, enzymes, nucleic acids etc. Natural endogenous substances or drugs may be effectors that occupy the effective surface of the targeting agent and affect the target positively or negatively. Computer aided drug molecule design and development studies are examined in two groups:

1. Based on effector (ligand) structure

   • Quantitative structure-activity relationships analysis (QSAR)

   • Pharmacophore analysis

2. Based on target structure

   • Molecular docking

   • Based drug design

It is aimed to interpret the structure of receptors by using the structure of molecules and acting on ligand structure. In method based on the target structure, it is aimed to design molecules that can act on the basis of the known receptor structure [6].

In summary, computational models can be used to simulate complex situations prior to testing in reality, allowing us to make these inevitable mistakes and helping us to successfully avoid their deleterious impacts of new proposed drugs.

4. In silico models

It is generally recognized that drug discovery and development are time and resources consuming. There is an ever-growing effort to apply computational power to the combined, chemical and biological space? in order to streamline drug design, development and optimization. Computer-aided or in silico design is being utilized to expedite and facilitate identification, optimize the absorption, distribution, metabolism, excretion and toxicity (ADMET) profiles and avoid safety issues. In silico modeling significantly minimizes the time and resource requirements of synthesis and biological testing. The aim is to enrich the group of molecules with the desired properties (active, drug-like, lead-like) and to eliminate those exhibiting unwanted properties (inactive, reactive, toxic, weak ADMET/pharmacokinetic profile).

The result is a compounds library and, by virtual screening using in silico methods, the number of molecules to be tested forward by experimental means, is considerably reduced. Structure-based library design is prejudiced by structural requirements for specific activity on a particular target and needs prior information of the target structure (e.g., X-ray or nuclear magnetic resonance). The goal is to select existing compound from libraries or to design compounds with three-dimensional complementarity (i.e., shape, size and physicochemical properties) to the target-binding site. New approaches can directly guide the design of virtual combinatorial libraries, which are first screened in silico for targeting complementarity, thus reducing the number of compounds will have to be synthesized and tested *in vitro*.

The "leading" compound has the desired pharmacolological or biological activity and represents the starting point to design other molecules with improuved properties/chemical parameters in terms of efficacy and pharmcokinetic profile, better candidates for future chemical synthesis and trials. When leading molecules have been identified, they have to be optimized in terms of potency, selectivity, pharmacokinetics and toxicology before they can become candidates for drug development. The early analysis in this respect is becoming common practice because the high overall attrition rate in drug discovery is affected the identification of compounds. Traditionally, therapeutics have been small molecules that fall within the Lipinski's rule of five [9]. From this point of view, hydrogen bonds, log P value, penetration into the targeting side can be mentioned. If the hydrogen bond donors are <5, the hydrogen receptors are <10, the relative molecular weight is <500 g/mol and the lipophilicity (log P) is <5, the compound will probably be orally bioavailable. The concepts of virtual library and virtual browsing have become an integral part of pioneering discoveries. In silico approaches significantly contribute to early pharmaceutical research and are especially important in target and lead discovery. The need has been clearly recognized and is expected to improve efficiency of drug design for timely adaptation and application of in silico models in pharmaceutical research [10]. European policy for the evaluation of chemicals (REACH: Registration, Evaluation, and Authorization of Chemicals) has been a strong advocate of alternative in silico methods of predictive evaluation of chemical toxicity in order to minimize animal testing and conserve time and resources [11].

5. Factorial Design for Drug Delivery

Design of Experiments (DoE) is defined as a planning strategy that will be carried out to obtain the information from the collected data effectively. It is a structural method used to determine the relationship between different factors (independent variable, input, process parameter, formulation component, etc.,) and their responses (dependent variable, response variable, output, product quality feature, etc.,). Also, this model is a mathematical model that correlates all the relevant factors and the results obtained against these factors. The results can be interpreted, predicted and the design space can be determined by optimization with this mathematical model. Systematic DoE approaches have advantages such as less experimental study, easier problem identification and prevention, any active agent adjuvant interaction and product performance to guarantee an effective formulation, and process optimization for good results in the scale up process.

An ideal drug form design should be depended on the understanding of the physicochemical and mechanical transformations of the materials that will eventually turn into the desired product. However, due to the diversity and complexity of the drug components, it is usually not fully understood. Factorial design with a systematic approach the product and production process can be understood in depth. In this way, a development approach can be provided which takes into account the variability of the inputs and other risks that may arise against product quality.

It is very important to obtain the basic knowledge of the study in order to produce as much information as possible with the right modeling. The statistical analysis is the first stage of experimental work before optimizing the formulation. Simple models are used in statistical screening. For example, linear models with only the main factor effects, or linear models, including binary interactions. In this way, the factors that have the most effect on the outputs are determined with the least number of tests possible. Factors with little or no significant effect can be displayed. In addition, by decreasing the number of factors, optimization design with a smaller number of attempts can be used.

The choice of DoE should be based on the number and type of factors to be investigated. For example, if the goal is only to reduce the number of factors and find a few factors that have the highest effect on the outputs, and if there are too many factors to be investigated, then the statistical elimination by constructing linear models can be selected. The results consist in lowering the number of attempts and evaluate only the main factor effects. The most preferred statistical screening methods in drug formulations are two-level partial full factorial design and Plackett-Burman design [12].

After statistical screening, response surface modeling (RSM) designs are started. The number of factors should be reduced by the statistical elimination design before the RSM design, so that the number of trials is not high and the statistical significance is important/relevant or other synonym and strong prediction models can be established. RSM is an approach where statistical and mathematical techniques are used together for the development and optimization of pharmaceutical processes. Includes modeling techniques used to determine the relationship between dependent variables and the independent variables that affect them.

RSM designs for drug formulations allow us to understand the relationship between factors and response variables, as well as factor interactions (synergistic effect of two or more factors), quadratic effects, and cubic terms. In this way, the optimum value ranges of the factors are provided. Process problems can be solved. Robust processes that are less sensitive to process variability can be developed.

Each additional experiments and sample analysis performed to product development in the pharmaceutical industry means that spending a lot of money, time and labor loss. The selection, implementation and interpretation of the appropriate factorial design that serves to reach the result accurately and rapidly is very important. Selecting the appropriate experimental design ensures that development studies are completed with a small number of trials. In order to optimize the process and formulation, mathematical models are described that best relationship between these critical factors and quality characteristics [13].

6. Computational models for radiopharmaceuticals

Computer models in the pharmaceutical industry is used to discover new drugs, to optimize of chemical processes and to design clinical trials. Accurate computational estimation of the responses to the treatments and clinical profiles of administration is of great importance for patients [14–19]. Also, it is very useful to help clinicians decide on the most effective and least toxic treatment available options, and is significant for researchers to selecte for *in vitro* and *in vivo* studies [20–22]. In addition, the computational prediction of drug responses can substantially contribute to preclinical studies, as in silico drug screening model. These tools can help researchers in the selection of candidate compounds in their research, and can be used to improve efficiency in experimental planning and to reduce costs [23–25]. Especially, computational estimation of drug responses in cancer disease involves significant research challenges. It is a biological challenge since cancer is a very heterogeneous and multifactorial disease. Furthermore, increasing the need for data integration, new technical questions arise from multiple sources such as the adjustment and normalization of data from multiple sources [14]. In the Oak Ridge National Laboratory, Snyder [26] the first mathematical model of radiopharmaceuticals was realized. In this design, the fractions of energies and amount of gamma and X-rays emitted from radiopharmaceuticals in the targeting tissue were used by Monte Carlo method [26]. Computational model supports the development of radiolabeled complex synthesis and coordination chemistry of radiopharmaceuticals by providing a better understanding of the physicochemical properties of molecular imaging agents. Combining experimental studies with computational study helps to define structure-activity relationships of radiopharmaceuticals and facilitates the rational design of new generation radiopharmaceuticals with improved properties. Francisco et al. [27] used different computational simulators to investigate the therapeutic potential of various radionuclides. These simulators are:

- Fast Monte Carlo damage formation simulator.

- Fast Monte Carlo excision repair simulator.

- Virtual Cell Radiobiology Simulator [27].

Fast Monte Carlo damage formation simulator can be used to estimate the types of DNA damage and post-irradiation efficiency. This method allows multiple data analyzes with multiple irradiation estimates to be collected as soon as possible [28, 29].

Fast Monte Carlo excision repair simulator can be used to estimate the occurrence, repair of DNA and correct repair results by mutation [27].

Virtual cell radiobiology simulator is a radiobiological model used to describe dose response relationship, damage production process and key repair mechanisms. These models often relate the dose rate to the cell's response to irradiation. Some of the current models include a repair-false-repair model, a fatal potentially fatal model, and two lesion kinetics [28].

In one study, the Monte Carlo method was used to assess the amount of radionuclide in animal models for preclinical testing of radiopharmaceuticals. In another study, this model predicted 3D images simulated with SPECT or PET for patient-specific radionuclide treatments [27, 28].

Computational methods allow quick and easy data collection. However, some models are based on available information and are evaluated according to this information and this imposes some restrictions. The used algorithms report an optimal ionization scenario to ionize the DNA in place of ineffective radionuclide biodistribution process that is obtained by *in vitro* and *in vivo* studies under difficult conditions. Thus, although the validation of the used simulators has been performed in selected irradiation scenarios and specific cellular populations, specifying these methods may be useful as a first step approach to large data sets to assist in the planning of *in vitro* and *in vivo* studies [29–33].

Kurniawan et al. [34] studied on radiopharmaceutical ligands and concrete examples of molecular docking. T3, 4BCPP is an imidazolylporphyrin derivative and has been used as a radioimaging agent for melanoma cancers. They designed new imidazolylporphyrin derivatives with better selectivity and higher affinity than T3, 4BCPP by using AutoDock 4.2. After that they develop a new radiopharmaceutical by using a radionuclide such as Technetium (Tc) for diagnostic and Rhenium (Re) for therapeutic purposes. They concluded that radiolabelled imidazolylporphyrin derivatives could be two potential candidate ligands for a melanoma radiopharmaceutical kit.

Chen et al. [35] assessed the effects of structural modification on the interaction of ^{125}I-labeled iodo Hoechst ligands and DNA. Also, they designed new analogs with specified distances between the Auger-electron-emitting ^{125}I atom and the DNA central axis by using computer-assisted molecular modeling software. This software program has been obtained the reactivity of newly designed radiolabelled molecules with their targeted DNA molecules by molecular modeling prior to their chemical synthesis.

El-Motaleb et al. [36] developed an easy method for radio iodination of propranolol with high percent labeling yield for the purpose of lung perfusion imaging. They used molecular modeling and docking studies to ensure the binding of the newly obtained radio iodination of propranolol to beta-2 adrenergic receptor and confirmed that radio iodination did not affect the binding of propranolol to beta-2 receptor by using molecular modeling.

7. Conclusion

Computational methodology provides some advantages such as creating time-dependent organ dose rate curves, making easier for researchers and clinicians to take the right choices. Also, these approaches give accurate and effective results and reduce the cost of research being useful to simulate complex situations before research, to avoid harmful/side effects. Furthermore, the radiopharmaceutical dosimetry estimates demonstrate large variation due to the patient's anatomical characteristics and computational model can be useful for obtaining personalized data. We believe that using these methods could enhance the personalization of dosimetry in nuclear medicine administration.

Author details

Emine Selin Demir, Emre Ozgenc, Meliha Ekinci, Evren Atlihan Gundogdu*,
Derya İlem Özdemir and Makbule Asikoglu
Radiopharmacy Department, Faculty of Pharmacy, Ege University,
Bornova, Izmir, Turkey

*Address all correspondence to: evren.atlihan@gmail.com

IntechOpen

References

[1] Ocak M, Beaino W, White A, Zeng D, Cai Z, Anderson CJ. Cu-64-labeled phosphonate cross-bridged chelator conjugates of c(RGDyK) for PET/CT imaging of osteolytic bone metastases. Cancer Biotherapy and Radiopharmaceuticals. 2018;**33**:74-83

[2] Wadsaka W, Mitterhausera M. Basics and principles of radiopharmaceuticals for PET/CT. European Journal of Radiology. 2010;**73**(3):461-469

[3] National Physical Laboratory. Measurement Good Practice Guide No 93. Protocol for Establishing and Maintaining the Calibration of Medical Radionuclide Calibrators and their Quality Control. London: HMSO; 2006

[4] Quality Assurance of Radiopharmaceuticals. Report of a Joint Working Party: The UK Radiopharmacy group and the NHS pharmaceutical quality control committee. Nuclear Medicine Communications. 2001;**22**:909-916

[5] Aşikoğlu M. In: Gürsoy A, editor. Radyofarmasötikler, Farmasötik Teknoloji Temel Konular Ve Dozaj Şekilleri. Vol. 9. İstanbul: Kontrollü Salım Sistemleri Derneği Yayını; 2004. pp. 399-407

[6] Aşikoğlu M, İlem Özdemir D. Radioimaging and diagnostic application. In: Senyigit T, Ozcan I, Ozer O, editors. Nanotechnology in Progress. İzmir: IConcept; 2012. pp. 160-173

[7] Brian J, Schmidt J, Papin A, Musante CJ. Mechanistic systems modeling to guide drug discovery and development. Drug Discovery Today. 2013;**18**(1):116-127

[8] Fernald GH. Bioinformatics challenges for personalized medicine. Bioinformatics. 2011;**27**:1741-1748

[9] Goodwin RJA, Bunch J, McGinnity DF. Mass Spectrometry Imaging in Oncology

Drug Discovery. In: Richard R. Drake, Liam A. McDonnell Editors. Advances in Cancer Research; 2013:133-171

[10] Michelson S, et al. Target identification and validation using human simulation models. In: León D, Markel S, editors. In Silico Technologies in Drug Target Identification and Validation. Vol. 6. CRC Press/Taylor & Francis Group; 2007;**50**(9):2278-2279

[11] Kapetanovic IM. Computer-aided drug discovery and development (CADDD): In silico-chemico-biological approach. Chemico-Biological Interactions. 2008;**171**(2):165-176

[12] Sahu AK, Jain V. Screening of process variables using Plackett-Burman design in the fabrication of gedunin-loaded liposomes. Artificial Cells Nanomedicine and Biotechnology. 2017;**45**(5):1011-1022

[13] Demir Ö, Aksu B, Özsoy Y. İlaç Formülasyonu Geliştirilmesinde Deney Tasarımı (DoE) Seçimi ve Kullanımı. Marmara Pharmaceutical Journal. 2017;**21**(2):216-227

[14] Azuaje F. Computational models for predicting drug responses in cancer research. Briefings in Bioinformatics. 2017;**18**(5):820-829

[15] Adams JU. Genetics: Big hopes for big data. Nature. 2015;**527**(7578):108-109

[16] Schmidt C. Cancer: Reshaping the cancer clinic. Nature. 2015;**527**(7576):10-11

[17] Rubin MA. Health: Make precision medicine work for cancer care. Nature. 2015;**520**(7547):290-291

[18] Kohane IS. Health care policy. Ten things we have to do to achieve precision medicine. Science. 2015;**349**(6243):37-38

[19] Baselga J, Bhardwaj N, Cantley LC. AACR cancer progress report 2015. Clinical Cancer Research. 2015;**21**(19):S1-S128

[20] Simon R. Drug-diagnostics co-development in oncology. Frontiers in Oncology. 2013;**3**:315

[21] Relling MV, Evans WE. Pharmacogenomics in the clinic. Nature. 2015;**526**(7573):343-350

[22] Aronson SJ, Rehm HL. Building the foundation for genomics in precision medicine. Nature. 2015;**526**(7573):336-342

[23] Boehm JS, Golub TR. An ecosystem of cancer cell line factories to support a cancer dependency map. Nature Reviews. Genetics. 2015;**16**(7):373-374

[24] Caponigro G, Sellers WR. Advances in the preclinical testing of cancer therapeutic hypotheses. Nature Reviews. Drug Discovery. 2011;**10**(3):179-187

[25] Klijn C, Durinck S, Stawiski E. A comprehensive transcriptional portrait of human cancer cell lines. Nature Biotechnology. 2015;**33**(3):306-312

[26] Snyder WS, Ford MR, Warner GG, Fisher HL. Estimates of Absorbed Fractions for Monoenergetic Photon Sources Uniformly Distributed in Various Organs of a Heterogeneous Phantom. New York, NY: Society of Nuclear Medicine; 1969. MIRD pamphlet no. 5

[27] Francisco DC, Liberala G, Alexandre A, Tavares S, Manuel RS. Comparative analysis of different radioisotopes for palliative treatment of bone metastases by computational methods. Medical Physics. 2014;**14**(3):191-199

[28] Semenenko V, Stewart RD. A fast Monte Carlo algorithm to simulate the spectrum of DNA damages formed by ionizing radiation. Radiation Research. 2004;**161**(4):451-457

[29] Sach RKS, Feld P, DJB E. The link between low-LET dose-response relations and the underlying kinetics of dam age production/repair/misrepair. International Journal of Radiation Biology. 1997;**72**(4):351-374

[30] Wesley EB. The Monte Carlo method in nuclear medicine: Current uses and future potential. Journal of Nuclear Medicine. 2010;**51**(3):23-27

[31] Stabin MG, Peterson TE, Holburn GE, Emmons MA. Voxel-based mouse and rat models for internal dose calculations. Journal of Nuclear Medicine. 2006;**47**:655-659

[32] Padilla L, Lee C, Milner R, Shahlaee A, Bolch WE. Canine anatomic phantom for preclinical dosimetry in internal emitter therapy. Journal of Nuclear Medicine. 2008;**49**:446-452

[33] Guerrero M, Stewart RD, Wang JZ, Li XA. Equivalence of the linear-quadratic and two-lesion kinetic models. Physics in Medicine and Biology. 2002;**47**(17):3197-3209

[34] Kurniawan F, Kartasasmita RE, Tjahjono DH. Computational study of imidazolylporphyrin derivatives as a radiopharmaceutical ligand for melanoma. Current Computer-Aided Drug Design. 2018;**14**(3):191-199

[35] Chen K, Adelstein J, Kassis AI. Molecular modeling of the interaction of iodinated Hoechst analogs with DNA: Implications for new radiopharmaceutical design. Journal of Molecular Structure: THEOCHEM. 2004;**711**(1-3):49-56

[36] El-Motaleb MA, Farrag AS, Ibrahim IT, Sarhan MO, Ismail MF. Preparation and molecular modeling of radioiodopropranolol as a novel potential radiopharmaceutical for lung perfusion scan. International Journal of Pharmacy and Pharmaceutical Sciences. 2015;**7**(8):110-116

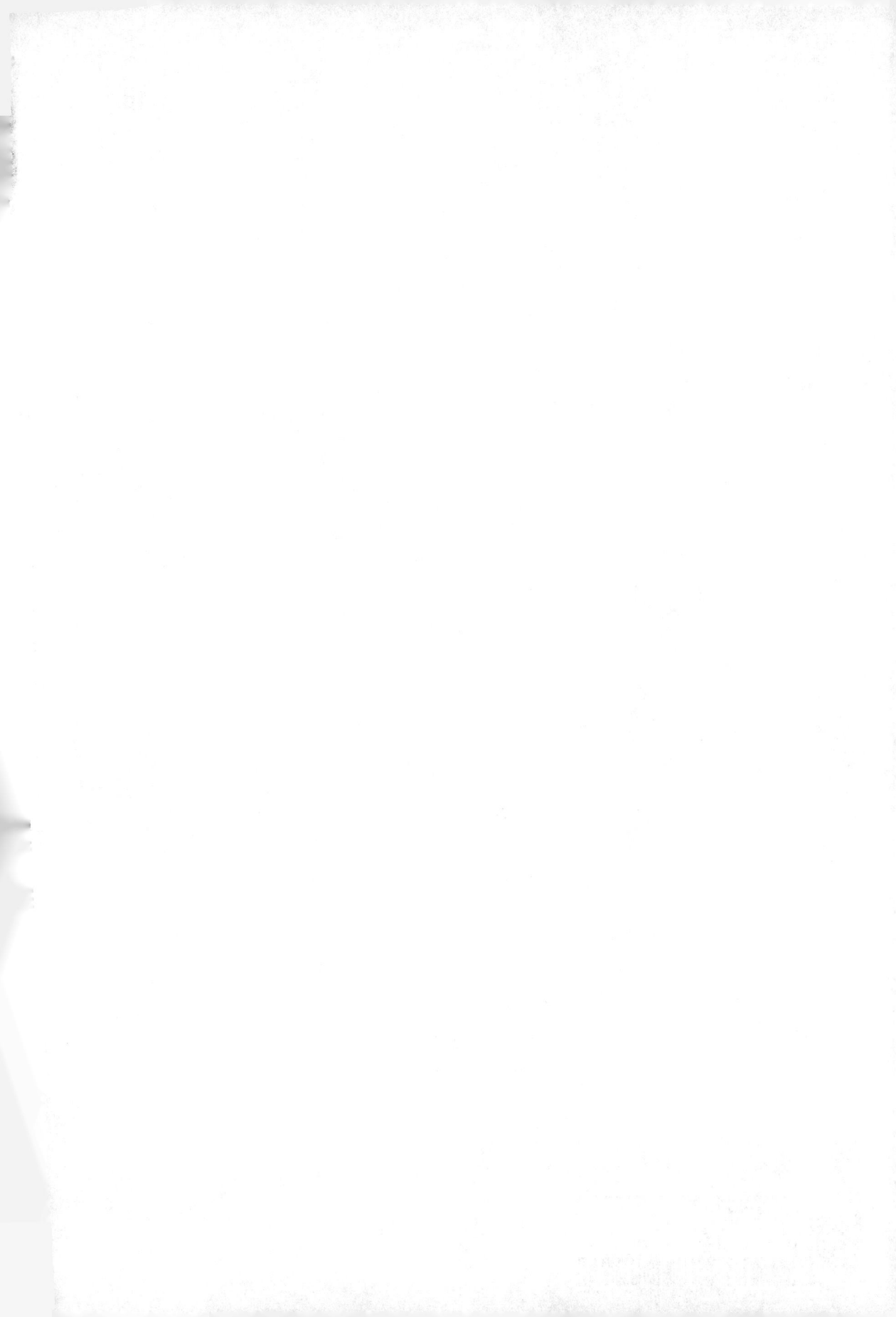